My Pinewood Kitchen

130+ Crazy Delicious, Gluten-Free Recipes to Reduce Inflammation and Make Your Gut Happy

Mee McCormick

Health Communications, Inc.
Boca Raton, Florida

www.hcibooks.com

Library of Congress Cataloging-in-Publication Data
is available through the Library of Congress

© 2020 Mee Tracy McCormick

ISBN-13: 978-07573-2352-2 (Paperback)
ISBN-10: 0-7573-2352-9 (Paperback)
ISBN-13: 978-0-7573-2353-9 (ePub)
ISBN-10: 0-7573-2353-7 (ePub)

Before beginning any new dietary plan, readers are encouraged to
consult with their current health provider.

HCI, its logos, and marks are trademarks of Health Communications, Inc.

Publisher: Health Communications, Inc.
          1700 NW 2nd Ave.
          Boca Raton, FL 33432-1653

Cover photo: Heather Muro
Cover design: Ted Raess
Interior photography: Heather Muro, Michael Bromley Jr., and Kirkland Pinkerton
Food stylists: Jake Stearns and Nicole Tracy
Interior design and formatting: Lawna Patterson Oldfield

Don't be distracted wondering where you will go,
but be present and grow where you are.

To everyone who helped me get where I am,
especially Lee, Bella, and Lola.

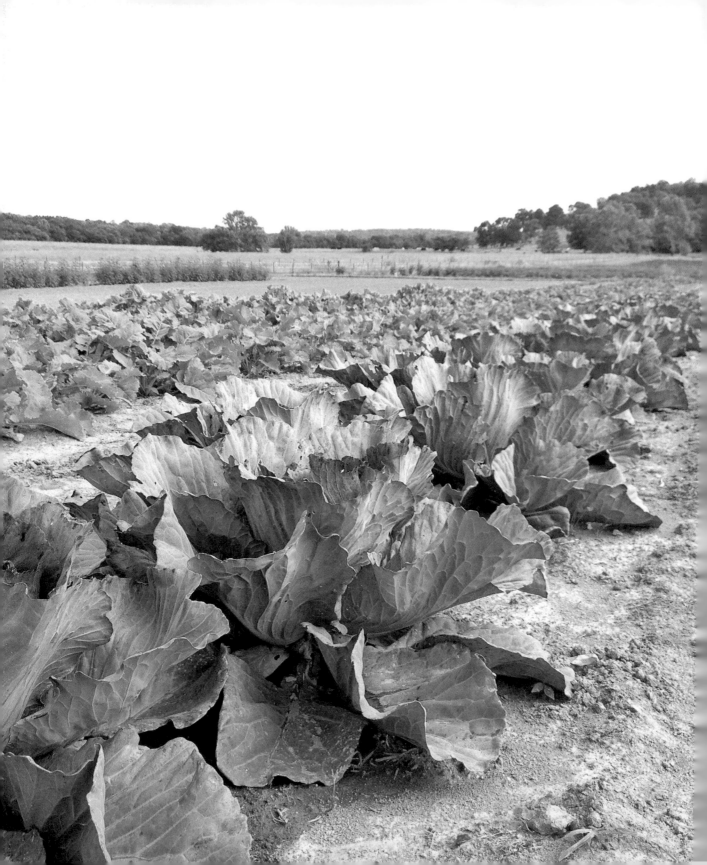

Contents

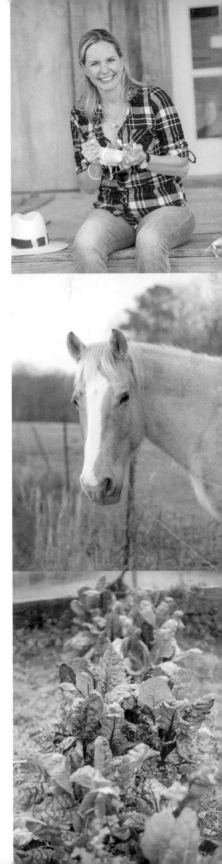

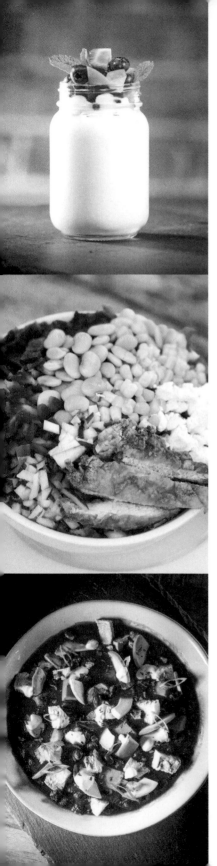

Veggies to Make Your Gut Happy

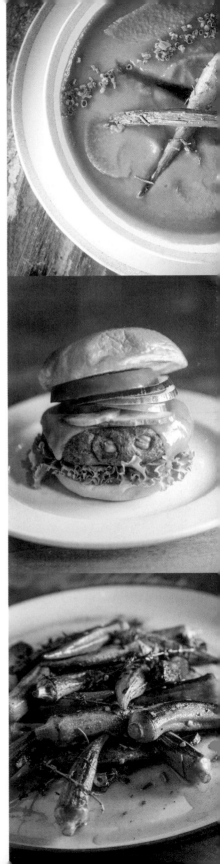

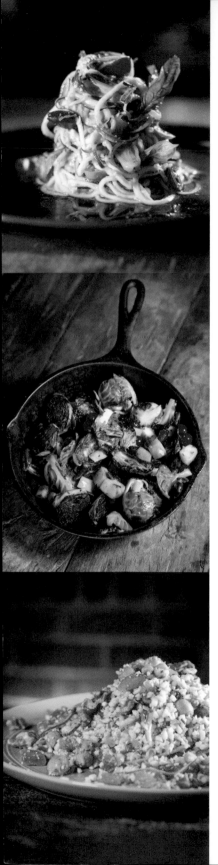

Glorious Gluten-Free Baking & Sweet Endings

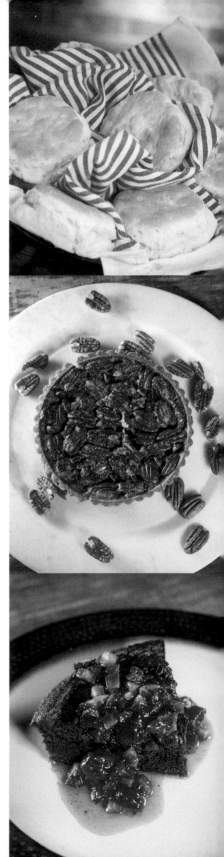

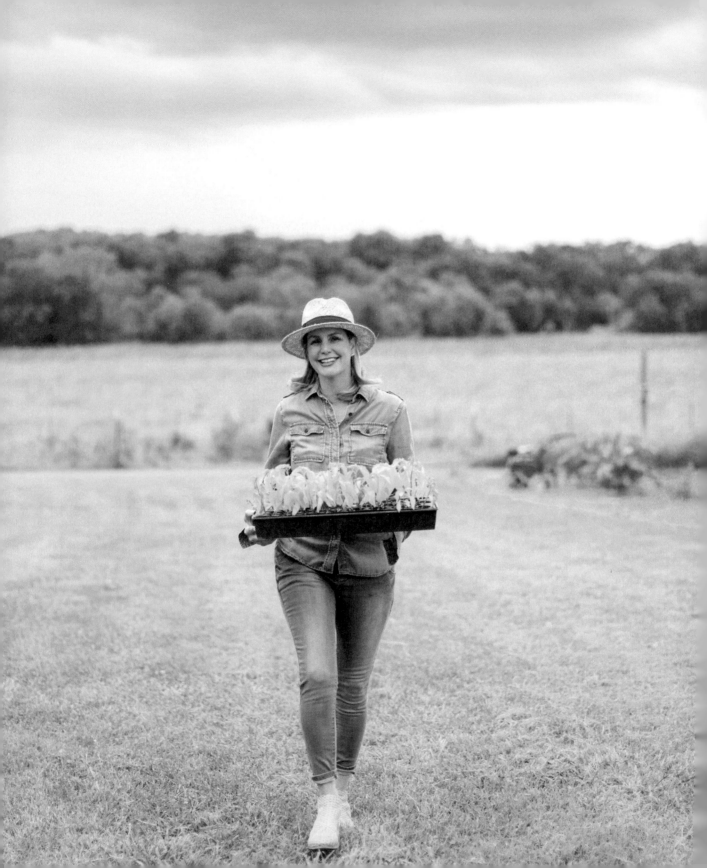

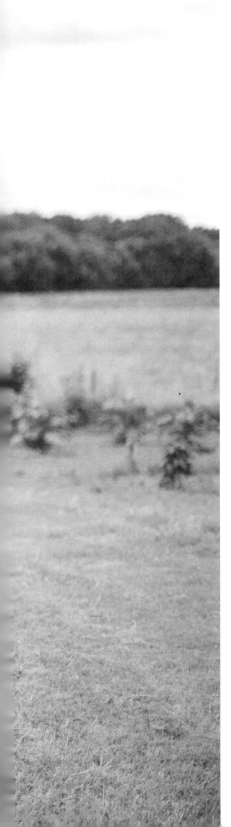

Foreword

I t is entirely possible that Mee McCormick is the coolest person on the planet. Who else could write a cookbook so inspiring, so informative, and so much fun that it's almost impossible to put down? And that's before you even get to her recipes, which are so delicious that it's practically a crime to eat anything else.

I first met Mee a couple of weeks after she gave birth to Lola, her youngest daughter. Suffering from ulcerations in her intestines and undiagnosed Crohn's disease, Mee was so frail and thin that baby Lola was practically bigger than she was. Only the fiercest mama could even have survived with no apparent hope in sight from the medical establishment. And survive Mee did. Even better, she has thrived, becoming one of the leading experts on how food can reduce inflammation and help heal us from the modern epidemics of autoimmune diseases and other health challenges.

Mee's journey from death's door to Pinewood Kitchen is a page turner. She became her own lab rat, learning how to cook in order to heal herself, and she became the best self-taught scientist I've ever met. I should know. I'm a pretty good scientist myself, with a doctorate from Harvard Medical School, although truth be told, my cooking is still in grade school.

As phenomenal as Mee is, none of us thrive alone. Her devoted husband, Lee, and their daughters, Bella and Lola, are quite the family. You'll enjoy the photos of them working in their organic gardens, cowboying on their grass-fed cattle ranch, and serving delicious food (and playing really great music) on the weekends in Pinewood Kitchen. At a time in history when just about everything seems to be falling apart, the McCormicks are living proof that we can all come together, help each other move forward, and have a fine time on the adventure—even when the going gets really rough.

So c'mon in to the Pinewood Kitchen and join the community. We all want to live well and give our families joy, health, and connection. That's what the McCormick clan is all about. And that's what Pinewood is all about, too. Bringing a community to life in a way that heals the heart, honors the land, and helps us remember that life is a beautiful gift.

—Joan Borysenko, Ph.D.
New York Times Bestselling Author

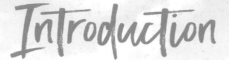

Introduction

Welcome to Pinewood, Y'all

The best part about life is what we can't see coming. The older I get and the more experiences I have, the better I am at trusting the unknown. I have struggled in my life with health and great loss. But what I've been given as a result of that loss and struggle is more than I could have dreamed, proving it happened *for* me, not *to* me. Never in a million years did I imagine I would end up in Pinewood, an hour's drive from Nashville, Tennessee, running Pinewood Kitchen & Mercantile with my husband, Lee, and our daughters, Bella and Lola. Our little restaurant on the farm has something for everyone, just like the recipes in this book. To understand how we arrived here, I hope you'll follow me down the road to Pinewood in Part One.

In Part Two, I'll share with you all the research I've discovered about how to keep our guts happy—and why our guts have *everything* to do with our health—from food allergies and intolerances to digestive disorders and even depression. I'm so excited to introduce you to our "gut homies," the helpful bacteria in our microbiome, and offer you tips on how to keep them healthy and happy through a diverse diet. You'll become an expert in how to stock your kitchen with foods that can help keep you clear of gut inflammation and digestive distress.

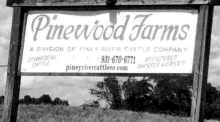

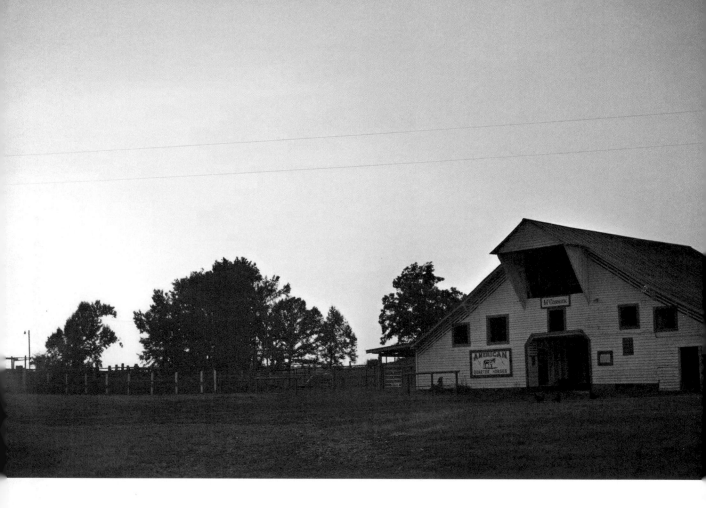

Then, in Part Three, I'll meet you in the kitchen with reimagined classic Southern recipes that will do your body good. They are all gluten free. Whenever possible, I include substitutions to make a dish dairy free, meat free, or grain free. You must be the judge of what's right for your body. For example, if you know you have an allergy to an ingredient or an intolerance, skip that recipe or experiment with a different ingredient that you know your body likes.

I hope this book leads you to find your own road to optimal gut health and that it inspires you to cook with an open mind and an open heart, experimenting with different flavors and foods for yourself and those who come to your table. Pinewood has led me to live with more empathy and kindness, showing me that our tiny little kitchen is leading the way with a new level of hospitality, and there isn't a better place to kick this off than in the warmhearted South.

Part One

The Long and Winding Road to Pinewood

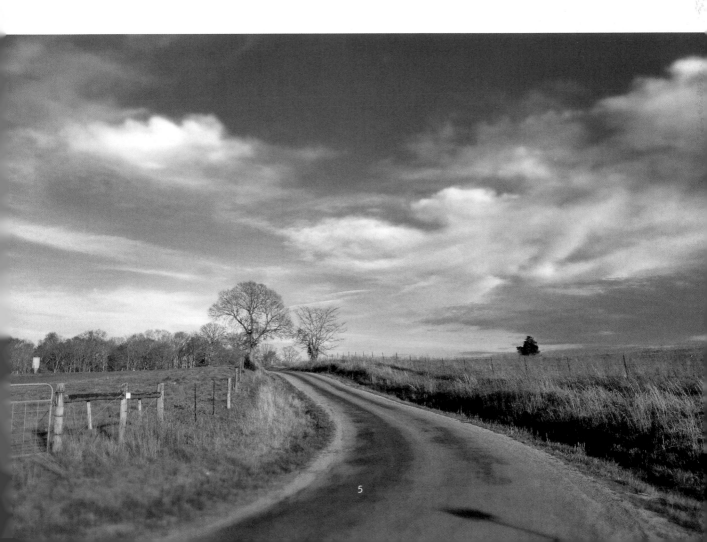

In the 1980s, I watched *A Coal Miner's Daughter* on my grandparents' old television set. While the credits ran, I said to myself, "I'm going to be like Loretta Lynn and go to fancy, important places." I decided that, like Loretta, I was gonna get outta those northern Appalachian Mountains.

And I did. I thought I needed to travel to BIG places to do BIG things, so I found myself moving all over the place. Starting in College Park, Maryland, I did a stint at the University of Maryland. Then I enrolled in school in New York City, where I had some big adventures, and then off I went to Los Angeles, where I really stepped into my adult self. From LA, I traveled back and forth to Tel Aviv, Israel, and learned to speak Hebrew. Sausalito, California, was my next stop, followed by Mexico City, and then Sayulita, Mexico, where I strengthened my Spanish skills and found one of the most important people in my life, Señora Gina, who, among many other things, made me the delicious, comforting soup I'll share with you in Part Three.

Of course, meeting my husband, Lee, has been my greatest blessing. He brought me to Pinewood, Tennessee, population 200. It's the smallest place I've ever lived and the BIGGEST thing I've ever done.

Pinewood isn't really a town. It's never been incorporated, but it's always been considered a community. It was first settled by Samuel Graham in the 1830s when he purchased the land. By the 1850s, the Pinewood Plantation and Pinewood community were well established. One thing that made Pinewood special was that Sam Graham believed in the equality of all men and did not support slavery. To pay his help equally, he created "Pinewood dollars." Pinewood was a completely self-

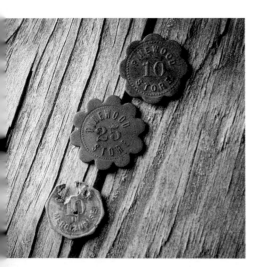

sustaining community. They grew hemp and made rope. They had their own mill on the river, acres of food, livestock, and a commissary store—the original Pinewood Store. At Pinewood's peak, close to 3,000 people were employed in the tiny community, and during the Civil War, some historians believe that at least 4,000 Confederate and Yankee soldiers passed through. Pinewood prospered and found its way until the late 1800s, when the land was divided and people moved away.

In the early 1990s, Lee and his stepfather, A. D. Davis, purchased the Pinewood Farm. They already knew a thing or two about livestock. You see, A. D., along with his brothers and father, are the founders of Winn Dixie, one of the first large grocery store chains in the United States. Known as "The Beef People," A. D. and his family transformed the beef industry by delivering cuts of meat directly to market. Lee was raised on ranches in Florida, Wyoming, and Colorado. Lee worked full time cowboying, and he currently runs the Piney River Cattle Company located on the old Pinewood Farm. Lee's dad had pioneer blood, too; his grandfather, B. B. McCormick, helped build the Flagler Railroad with Henry Flagler and was instrumental in building Jacksonville Beach, Florida.

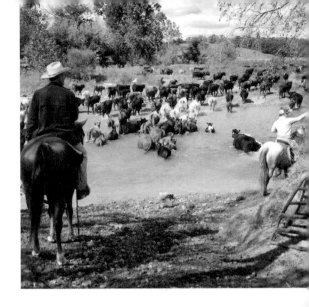

In the 1990s, Lee went to treatment for addiction issues and, in the process, reconnected with his spirit. He had such a profound experience that he built The Recovery Ranch in Pinewood, a residential treatment facility located where Sam Graham had built the tiny village of Pinewood. (Interesting fact is that when the Grahams ran Pinewood, it was a dry community—no alcohol.) While Lee was running the facility, I was living in Hollywood, working as an assistant stylist,

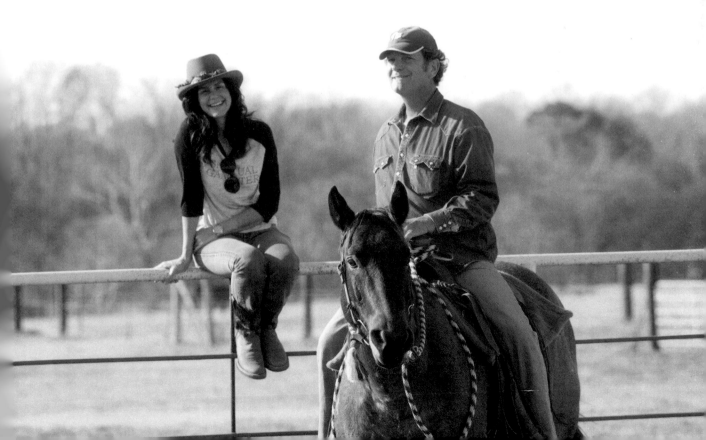

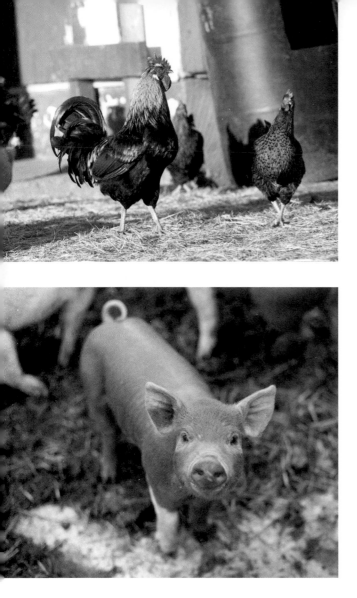

trying to make it as a writer and bartending at night. Close mutual friends who thought we'd hit it off introduced Lee and me via telephone. (These were the days before text messages and video chat.) We talked on the phone for months before we met.

On my first visit to Pinewood to meet Lee in person, I thought it was the most beautiful place I'd ever been. I just had no idea what in the world I would do there. I'd been living a fast and busy life in the city and felt I would struggle on the ranch. Fortunately, I didn't need to decide because Lee's work brought him to Malibu for part of the year. So, after we married, we celebrated living on the farm *and* on the beach.

When I met Lee, my digestive problems were part of the package. I'd lived with chronic pain, bloating, and occasional partial bowel obstructions for years before meeting him. My relationship with food had always been tricky. At birth, I was diagnosed with an intussusception, meaning my intestines collapsed inside themselves. Years later, I found out this was due to an ulceration I was born with. I immediately had a few inches of my small intestines cut away, but not before being baptized—the odds of my surviving back in the day were slim. I survived the surgery, but as a child, I struggled to digest many foods, and as a result, I was a pretty scrawny kid. In high school, my nickname was Cricket. I had food allergies, but no one paid much attention to them. Dairy was one of them, but my momma was a single parent and I had to eat what she fixed, which was minimal. She had Crohn's disease, and when she was super sick, she couldn't get up off the floor to cook or go to work. She spent a lot of time in the hospital during my childhood.

Food Stamps, Fish Sticks, and Missing My Momma

Food stamps became a major part of our fabric. My sister and I managed the kitchen, which meant Cheerios for dinner lots of nights. Chipped ham sandwiches on white bread with ketchup were downright fancy. Thankfully, my grandparents lived a couple of hours away in the northern Appalachian Mountains, and they took us for holidays and breaks, feeding us my grandmother's native Italian cuisine. (Pasta and tomato sauce will always be my comfort food.)

Sadly, my momma passed away when I was eighteen years old. I moved into the world with a dedication to live my best life. I did everything my mother didn't do. I waited to get married and have kids, I attended a university, and I traveled extensively and tried my best to create a big life. What I didn't do was change the culture of my gut (which I'll talk about in Part Two), so I was suffering much like my mother had.

After giving birth to our second daughter, Lola, I was rail thin. I couldn't eat much of anything. Even drinking water brought me to my knees with pain. Looking into my little girls' eyes, I saw the reflection of my own six-year-old self and knew I had to change my path. But how? Lee and I continued the hunt for an answer, visiting every doctor we could who might have an inkling of what to do to help me.

Lee's projects in Malibu ended, and we found ourselves living in the Mexican jungle. (How we got there is another story entirely.) I dedicated myself to writing, and Lee bounced back and forth between the ranch in Nashville and the jungle with the girls and me.

During a trip to Los Angeles to visit friends, I'd undergone yet another round of tests led by a young inquisitive doctor who was determined to figure out what was wrong. One day in the jungle, my cell phone rang, and Dr. Hunt-For-It was on the line in a tizzy: "Mee, you have to get out of the jungle now," he urged. "You are in danger of catching bad bacteria, typhoid, hepatitis, or worse, your intestines could rupture and kill you at any time. You need a hospital." Whoa! Apparently, a previous camera test that I'd undergone with another doctor showed that I had an ulceration the *total* circumference of my small intestines. Dr. Missed-It hadn't noticed it, but my new doctor had.

That phone call changed the direction of my life—and ultimately saved it.

Finding My Way Around the Kitchen

We packed as fast as we could and returned to Nashville and the ranch. I went to see a couple of doctors, and the only option was medicine to reduce the inflammation in my intestines and possible surgery. I knew I wouldn't survive the side effects of the medicine, and I could barely swallow the pills. I prayed about it. I heard guidance in the form of: "What's in it?" I took that to mean my food, since the only thing touching the lining of my intestines was what I ate.

Up until then, my idea of home cooking was purchasing mainly processed foods and serving them along with salads and fruits, thinking I was cooking healthy for my family, but now I knew that wasn't the case. So I connected with a woman who taught me about macrobiotics, and I found my way around the kitchen. However, the macrobiotic diet was too limiting, and I knew there had to be more ways to wellness. With some detective work, I discovered that I had many food allergies and sensitivities, which led me to master allergy-friendly cooking. I'm happy to say that a year after taking my kitchen back, I found digestive relief and the ulceration had healed.

I knew there were millions of people like me, searching for relief while being super intimidated by the kitchen, so I decided to write about my food journey. We were living in LA at the time for one of Lee's projects, so I enrolled in a professional culinary program there that focused on French and American classics. I thought the chefs teaching the courses would love to know how I swapped out ingredients, but NOPE—apparently, classic culinary school is just about the classics. They were right; I was there to learn from them, and I needed to. I was unable to taste most of what we made each day, so I'd run home and "Mee-ify" it—challenging myself to re-create dairy-free, gluten-free versions of the dishes.

It Gets Better . . .

I finished the culinary program as well as my first book, *My Kitchen Cure*. Right after my book's release, I was contacted by *The Better Show*. They invited me to be on regularly. I knew that anything I did with my newfound wellness must be connected to my service to others, so I agreed. The moment I set foot in their New York City studio, I knew I belonged. The cast, the crew, and the guests felt familiar and comfortable. Being on the show was fulfilling, but I had never been away from Lee and the girls for very long, so the experience was also challenging.

Soon, my cooking spots were the number-one requested segments. The way I was swapping ingredients and making over classic recipes meant that the Heartland of America, their market for the show, was paying attention and they, too, wanted to find ways to make changes in their kitchens. I wasn't alone in my kitchen and neither were they. The show ran for two more seasons, and I loved being a part of it. When it ended, my heart was sad, and I prayed for another path and another opportunity to serve.

When Lee finished his project in LA, we decided to move back to Pinewood. The girls were getting older, and we wanted them to have a tighter connection with the farm.

One day, after a trip to New York City post-show, I was having a bad bout of digestive issues. I had eaten at a restaurant before boarding the flight, and even though I told the waiter I couldn't eat gluten, it still found its way onto my plate. I was down for the count. I barely made it off the plane without an intestinal explosion! When Lee and the girls picked me up, I was green and sweating, hoping I could hold it together until we reached the farm.

As I stepped off the curb at passenger pickup, Lee jumped out and loaded my belongings, and Lola climbed into my lap (*Ouch, not my lap!*). As we pulled away, Lola announced, "Mommy, Daddy bought the Pinewood Store! You got your own restaurant!"

A restaurant? I didn't know whether to hit my husband or jump out of the moving car, but I was too weak for either.

The Reluctant Restauranteur

Lee and I had discussed buying the Pinewood Store for a while, but I didn't think he would actually do it. I'd worked in kitchens most of my life, but running one scared me. It was one thing to write a blog, take pictures in my home kitchen, cook on TV, and even write a book. But it was another thing to run a real food kitchen, manage the farm, and keep up with managing my health and kids.

In truth, I didn't think I could do it—not physically, intellectually, or emotionally. A restaurant of my own was out of my lane, and I knew I'd get run off the road. I had a list of why this negative belief was in place: When I was in first grade, my parents divorced, and I didn't learn to read until the end of second grade. I always felt less intelligent than my peers. In high school, our life was so challenging at home that no one asked me how I was doing academically, so I just scooted my way through. After my momma's death, I returned home and ran into an old teacher who asked me how I was. When I told him I was taking classes at the University of Maryland, he gasped and said, "Oh, man, you'll never pull that off." Adding to the list was a past boyfriend who always commented on how funny and creative I was, but insisted I could never be good at business because I wasn't *that* kind of smart. Regardless of how this belief system was created, I now believed it. And this negative belief had me shaking in my boots.

My sweet grandmother (my momma's momma) was staying with us at the farm. Whenever she heard me grumbling about the purchase of the Pinewood Store, she'd say, "Well maybe it's God's plan. You can't choose where you are going to serve; he does. Just wait and see." So I waited, but all I could see was failure.

On New Year's Eve 2014, we were having a big Cattle Company Christmas party down in our cookhouse, where we prepared food for our hardworking crew daily. The night of the party, the previous owner of the Pinewood Store stopped by with the papers for us to sign. I swear I saw pure relief on his face as Lee shook his hand. If he caught a glimpse of mine, he would have seen dread and fear, and he knew why—he'd lost money owning the Pinewood Store, and he knew how tough it was going to be for us.

The last thing I said to Lee before falling asleep that night was, "I'm not having anything to do with this, so please don't ask me to."

The following week, I met with a semi-local good-ole-boy chef from Nashville. What I mean by "good-ole-boy chef" is that he was from the old-school world of cooking. Because he was older, he unequivocally saw a professional kitchen as a man's world. Lee and this dude had made a plan that he would run the restaurant and they'd partner up. I was meeting him because I was having a hard time with our name being attached to a restaurant where they served sub-par food. My plan was to meet with the chef, hear his ideas, and slip out the back door—free of the store and any guilt I had.

As I entered the store, I was blown away. They'd salvaged all the materials from the farm and from the old buildings. I ran my hand over the counter, which was made of bricks from the original commissary Pinewood Store; I gazed up at the reclaimed beams and weathered wood that had held strong since the 1850s. The old was meeting the new. They'd laid the most beautiful hardwood floors, and the bathrooms looked amazing, too. I was in awe of the natural beauty and the history.

Good-ole-boy chef was there waiting for me. We sat down, and he began by telling me what he wanted to do with the menu and the place in general—he wanted to use disposable plastic tableware and feature a simple menu with cheap food to make the quickest profit. When I mentioned using fresh green beans and produce from the farm, he dismissed me, saying that canned food was quicker and cheaper. "Besides, that's what the locals are accustomed to," he added.

I asked him about the oils he'd cook with and what he'd use in the fryer. He said that corn, soy, and vegetable oil had the best price point and usually had an anti-foaming agent and preservatives (aka chemicals), which would extend the life of the oil so we'd only have to change the oil every couple of weeks. My stomach was turning just thinking of eating something out of that fryer!

In addition to the gnarly fryer, my problem with corn oil and vegetable oil is that it's heavily processed and it can be cut with cottonseed oil, which isn't a food—it's not even regulated by the FDA. Plus, it's one of the crops that contains the most pesticides on the planet. Cotton, when digested, can cause intestinal inflammation even for healthy people, which explains why we sometimes feel bloated after we've eaten fried food from a restaurant. Put that kind of oil in a fryer and heat it up, and you've got chemical stew. As for anti-foaming agents, those are some of the same chemicals found in our gas tanks out in front of the store. I didn't want to eat that, and I was sure no one in Pinewood would, either.

Then I dug deeper, asking how he felt about food allergies and supporting people with them. He shook his head. He explained that most people weren't interested in eating gluten free, and only a few people seemed to have "real" food allergies any way. It was pretty much nonexistent for his kitchen protocol.

My plan to stay quiet went out the window. The floodgates opened, and all the knowledge I'd gained while learning how to cook came gushing out. I let him know what type of oil is best for the fryer—non-GMO rice bran oil—and why it was important to avoid any other added chemicals and to change the oil every four days. He shook his head no. I told him I thought it was best to only use olive oil to sauté with and to make his own ketchup with umeboshi vinegar because it's alkaline, aids in digestion, and helps with gas and bloating (not to mention that he could control the added sugar). I also told him that using disposable tableware was harmful to the environment.

It was obvious I was getting on his nerves like a gnat at the dinner table, and he was trying to compose himself and not swat me away. He looked at me with smug eyes, leaned in, and spoke to me in a voice used to correct a child—just enough condescending inflection that I knew he thought I was an idiot. Yet his Southern accent was smooth, and as he spoke, he grinned a smile of *Ain't you sweet.*

"That all sounds great. I'm sure you have a lot of blog tips for housewives wanting to run a healthier kitchen, and I bet your homemade ketchup is great at home. However, I have been running restaurants in these parts since before you were born and making your own ketchup is too time-consuming. Rice bran oil—I ain't never heard of it, and you'll go broke changing the oil even once a week. Plus, you have to know your audience—folks in these parts don't want any of your California food. I know what they want. I don't think you need to worry about any of this—I got it all covered."

There was nothing left for me to say. I simply smiled a Southern ladylike smile and pushed my chair away from the table. I shook his hand and said, "I see you do."

I got in my car and drove the 45 miles back to our city house. Know my audience—for sure I did! I knew that regular folks wanted to spend money on real food and wanted to feel good when they left a restaurant, and I knew that regular folks wanted to eat food out of a freshly changed fryer. I knew what people wanted—just like me, they wanted to make better choices and still enjoy their favorite recipes. I started to have what I can only explain as a conversation with my Higher Self:

Mee: Seriously, why did I even bother meeting with that guy?

Higher Self: Because it matters what type of food he cooks and the ingredients.

Mee: Not really. I'm just going to fade into the background and mind my own business. I won't eat there, and I won't tell anyone we own it.

Higher Self: No, you've got to get yourself into the mix. How can you allow this chef to serve processed, fake food when you have an abundance of real, living foods on the farm?

That night, Lee asked how my meeting with good-ole-boy chef went. I answered, "Fine. Did y'all sign a contract yet?"

"No," he replied. "We're meeting tomorrow to talk about it."

With that, I reached over to my nightstand, picked up my phone, and sent good-ole-boy chef a text:

It was lovely to meet with you today. After our conversation, I am completely inspired. I have decided that I will be running the Pinewood Kitchen, and I will also be the head chef. We will no longer need your services. By the way, your meeting tomorrow with Lee is canceled.

In twelve years of my relationship with Lee, I had never stepped up and taken control of something the way I had that night. And yet, as soon as I hit Send, I wanted to smack myself. What in the hell was I thinking? Who was that sending such a text? I didn't know how to run a restaurant, a line (the kitchen space where they do the cooking), order inventory, or any of that, and I didn't know anyone who could teach me. I went to sleep praying I hadn't made a huge mistake.

Follow the Pinewood Country Road

There I was feeling like Dorothy lost in Oz—with no idea how I'd crash-landed in Pinewood—and hoping to collect the characters who could help me turn Pinewood into Emerald City.

I put an ad on Craigslist for a chef, and I reached out to Frank, a restaurant kitchen manager I'd met while selling our produce at a farmers' market in the city. I convinced Frank to come on as a consultant and help me set up my kitchen. With his guidance, I bought all the kitchen equipment, ordered stainless-steel tableware, and was introduced to Restaurant Depot—the mecca of restaurant supply stores.

Ebenezer, the first chef to answer my ad, was the first guy I hired. He was a semi-recent culinary graduate, working in hotel catering. He was young, hungry, very hairy, honest, deeply Christian, and a bit rigid. He knew some things, but together, we would learn a lot. He stayed with me for the first year. My sister, Nicole, stepped in after the first six months. She'd been helping build the gardens and was hesitant to join me in the kitchen (she was also intimidated by what the demands of restaurant life would bring), but she hopped on the line and soon became my right hand. The two of us basically built Pinewood together. Next came Miss Tina, Steff, Darcy, Gail, Mario, Kenzie, Sara, Chris, Michael, Kayla, Andrew, Caitlin, and Kris. Together we got the kitchen up and running with smoothness and consistency. It wasn't a *Mee* thing; it was a *we* thing.

And while the kitchen was in great shape, ordering food was a challenge. In *My Kitchen Cure,* I wrote about all the issues with eating in restaurants, such as the fryer oil and the hidden ingredients in food. Now I had to walk *My Kitchen Cure* talk, and it wasn't turning out to be so easy. The beef and pork would come from our farm; I'd get the chicken from the Amish, and they could supply eggs if we ran out. For years, we'd worked with Jeff Poppin, The Barefoot Farmer, who helped us grow our biodynamic produce gardens, so whatever we couldn't grow, we'd procure from him. But there were things we needed, like buns and bread, dried goods, cheeses, and more, that we didn't grow and needed to source. Unfortunately, in this remote country community, food-service delivery barely existed.

I had a meeting with the local representative from Sysco, which is the world's largest broadline food distributor, and she was super kind. I gave her a list of the goods I needed, and she hunted for them, but I wasn't like any client she'd ever had. I wanted to know what every ingredient was, if they'd been manufactured for food-allergy sensitivity, and whether it was GMO or, if possible, organic. This got tricky, so Phil, a regional director, stepped in to help me. He'd recently changed his food intake as a result of heart issues and totally supported what I was doing in Pinewood. It took extra effort on his part to contact the suppliers and dig deep to get me all the answers I was looking for, but he got them. Pinewood still enjoys a fantastic relationship with Sysco today.

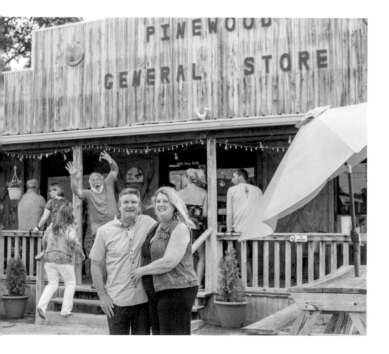

Opening Day

Not once during the process of setting up Pinewood was I concerned about who would come to eat there. When I have a task before me, that's what I focus on—not the outcome or grandiose fantasies. I just keep my head down and create. Our kitchen was stocked, and our cooks were in place. Our county was hosting their annual Arts & Agriculture Tour, and we were on the list. Folks would be able to tour our farm and then have lunch in the restaurant. I thought we might get a few tables and they would serve as practice for our kitchen. I had no idea how to cook for a "guess amount" of customers. I didn't even know what it meant to create food in volume.

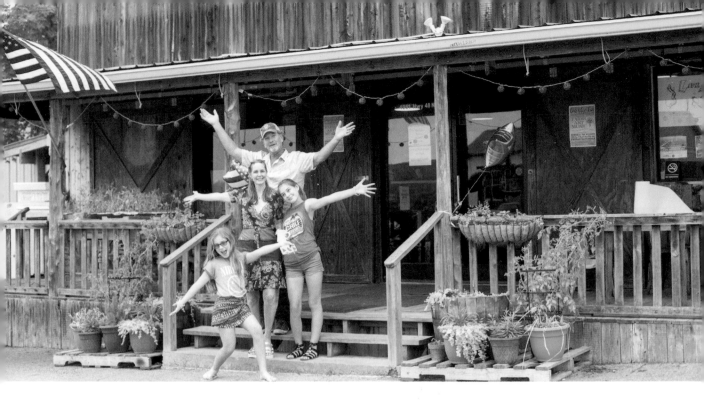

We rolled back the wooden doors to find a line of folks waiting to come in to eat. Within moments, it was mayhem. Every seat in the house (seventy of them) was taken. The kitchen was cranking and so was the chaos. I was jumping between the line and the floor, getting drinks, taking orders, cooking, plating, serving, bussing, sweeping, and stocking. Of course, our line wasn't functioning at its full potential, and we were drowning. Mistakes were flying and apologies flowing. Regardless, the folks kept coming in.

I had my own learning curve, starting with what I wanted to serve our guests. I thought I'd make the menu each day depending on what we had from the farm. I also didn't want to sell burgers every day. I thought everyone would want to eat lotus root soup, crispy tofu, burdock kinpira, and lovely greens and salad. NOT!

On opening day, most people wanted burgers and fries. Of course, I ran out of burgers. So, I introduced my rural community to falafel, a traditional Mediterranean chickpea burger. They ate it up, and the next day a couple of folks came in asking, "Ms. Mee, you got any more of that full-on awful burger left?" I was like, "What? My burger is awful?" Then, once they explained, I figured out they were asking about the *falafel* burger, not the *full-on awful* burger!

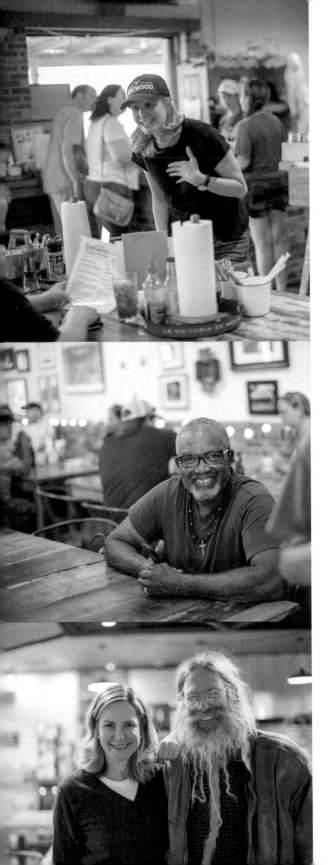

I did what many wellness food chefs and regular folks do when they get well or make a major change—I thought everyone should do it my way. Fat chance, and boy was I living from an arrogant place. Everyone has to find their own way, and I was about to learn that from my customers and my community.

Give 'Em What They Want— with a Healthy Twist

Pinewood began to shift when I started listening more and more to what people wanted to eat. I knew they wanted the hamburgers and fries. I was cranking that out like crazy. But I also found out they wanted soup, and so I began to master their favorite flavors while adding in superfood ingredients, and we were selling out. In fact, we sold so much that we started canning soups to sell and folks were calling ahead on the hottest summer days to find out what soup we had and if we'd canned any to go.

Soup is a great way to start when eating healthier because you can modify soups into powerhouse meals. I add nuts, mushrooms, probiotic miso pastes, and bone broths. For my vegans, I made a dashi seaweed broth or a mushroom veggie stock. Every server needed to know the ingredients so that they could educate the table. It was working. People were trying things they would never try before, and I was having a food epiphany: Serve people comfort food with a healthy twist and keep it delish. My cooking skills were expanding, and so was my point of view. I was truly becoming an inclusive chef.

I was learning that what people want is an *inclusive* table. Customers want a table where they can get a burger and fries and their child with a food allergy can safely eat without getting "glutened" or being given a stink eye from a waiter who finds food allergies annoying because it slows down the line and makes the chef cranky. They want to know that the place they are dining at is serving clean food. It's no longer just coastal hippies wanting organic food; deeply seated Southerners are also conscious of the environment. I was seeing that our customers needed to have a relationship with where our food comes from, and the people who are growing it and raising it matters greatly to these country folks. They'd mainly grown up on farms and craved that old-school connection at the table. I now know that people want to eat better-quality food and want to eat for wellness. People were loving that Pinewood was serving Southern food that wasn't sending folks home loaded and bloated.

The New Hospitality

I almost never eat out. I have food allergies, and often my choices on the menu are so slim I might as well just have water. There's always that side-eye question, "Is this an allergy or a preference?" If someone wants something gluten free, it should be handled with respect and hospitality. Because if someone says, "I'd like gluten *free*," that means *free of gluten*—not that they can have food with a few traces of gluten.

In Pinewood, we have a system. No buns on the grill; no cheese melted on the grill. All burgers and grilled

19

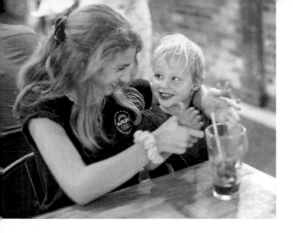

chicken go on individual trays, and the bun and cheese are heated and melted in the oven. Clean gloves are used on everything that's handled, and we use clean knives and separate cheese and sauce for gluten-free pizza—easy.

For the alpha-gal syndrome (a tick bite that leads to red meat allergy), we use a clean cast-iron skillet to cook chicken so that it isn't exposed to beef or pork. We keep the fryer 100% gluten free by cutting our potatoes by hand and we keep it pork/beef free. Any breaded food is hand breaded and gluten free. We have a separate station for gluten-free sandwiches and burgers. We always have vegan gluten-free salad dressings, including our ranch dressing. We use a soy-free miso paste in our soups. If someone has a legume allergy or nut allergy, we are prepared. The most important aspect is that everyone who works in the restaurant—from dishwasher to server—knows what's in the food and can serve customers with care and knowledge.

Our level of care spread like wildfire through middle Tennessee: If you have food allergies, you can eat in Pinewood. Next thing I knew, we had people driving for hours to eat with us. Sometimes they'd have a list of what they couldn't have, and we would create a meal just for them. My cooks and chefs were in alignment with me. We were training everyone in the kitchen how to be conscious of others, serving up consideration and empathy with each plate that came out of our kitchen.

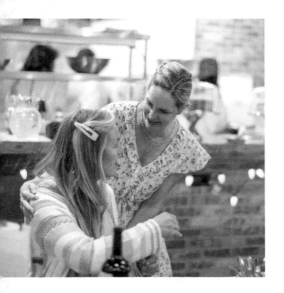

But there was also plenty of pushback. A couple of employees came with the building, and I wanted to keep them employed. Plus, many of the people I hired had never heard of gluten free, vegan, probiotic foods, macrobiotic, Paleo, or keto. Lots of people thought anything "organic" made food taste weird and didn't want to try it. I spent loads of time explaining it all, knowing that it was up to me to educate them and guide them. Everyone was on a journey of transformation.

However, one particular employee, a sweet young woman, disappeared one day in the middle of a busy Sunday brunch. Thinking she'd been kidnapped, I went on a mad hunt through Pinewood to look for her. Later I found out that she thought she'd served a gluten-free person gluten by mistake and freaked out. I couldn't believe it. I never imagined someone would walk out on a shift, and I never thought she would be so very upset and think she could have killed a person with gluten. I did miss Ms. Joey, but I knew the position was too much for her.

The good news was that I knew I had something special in Pinewood—my caring for others' wellness had attracted a staff that cared, too. Not only do we have staff, we have volunteers: Miss Lesa, Miss Donna, Glinda, and Sherry. When they see cars in the parking lot, they come in to wash dishes, work the register, and bus tables—for free—as they believe in the goodness of Pinewood and want to see it succeed. What's more, it's shocking how many people drive to Pinewood to share their stories of illness and healing via food. I think people come to see me play the tambourine and dance around the kitchen because they know how hard it was for me to climb up off the floor and now feel so good again. They see themselves in me, and maybe the Universe is using me to inspire hope.

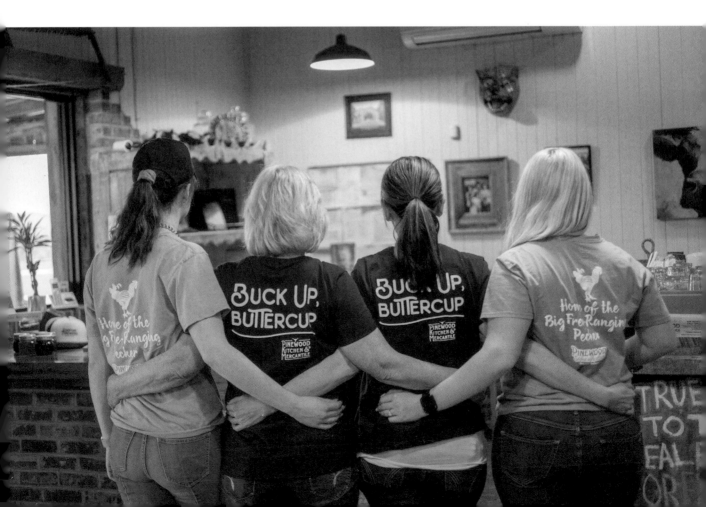

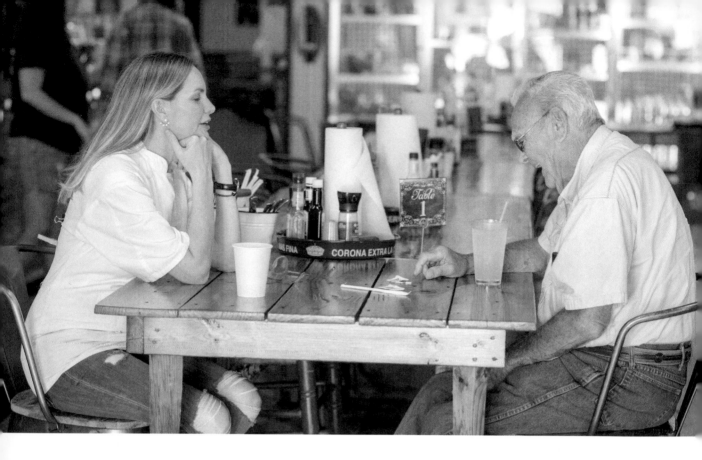

Creating a Culture

Now that I've been running Pinewood for almost five years, I see what I was really afraid of—failing as a leader. I'd only worked in kitchens run by tough men or women. The chef was the boss, the line yelled at the servers, intensity was key, and "agro" energy ricocheted off the pots and pans. Getting the food bought as cheap as could be and cranked out of the kitchen as fast as possible was the goal of all restaurant owners and chefs.

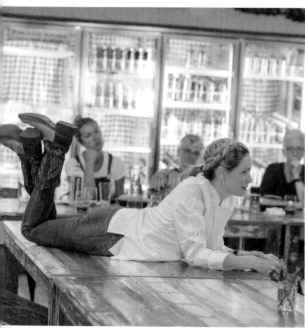

I'd never worked in a kind kitchen. Even as a kid, my momma and grandmother worked from a place of anger. The harder they cleaned, the crabbier they got. When I had kids, I saw myself reenacting what I was raised in. I thought, *Oh man, this is crazy—I have a beautiful house, I have wonderful kids. Why am I crabby when I clean? Why am I complaining about cooking every night when I'm so very blessed to have food to cook?*

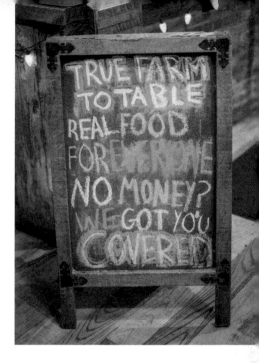

So, I shifted my point of view. I now find kitchen work and housework to be meditative. My sister, Nicole, and I both worked through this together in Pinewood. As the eldest sibling, she took on the weight of my mother's burdens. She ran the house when my momma was sick or in the hospital. She raised my brother and me when my momma died. In truth, she didn't have much of a childhood, and therefore her inheritance of my playfulness passed her by.

I can't even begin to tell you the healing Pinewood Kitchen has given my sister and me. We watched our momma suffer, not being able to eat or provide food for her kids, and we were helpless, hungry children. To be placed in a position to serve others real food that is mindful of their needs has been an incredible blessing bestowed upon us. From the day we opened, I implemented a policy that we feed everyone, regardless of their ability to pay. If there had been a Pinewood Kitchen when I was a little girl, I wouldn't have gone as hungry, and my momma could have eaten without pain.

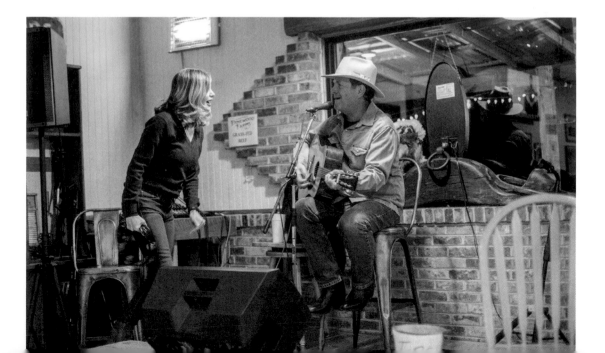

Running Pinewood meant our entire family had to join in. My daughter, Lola, at eight years old became the best cashier in town and my other daughter, Bella, could run the entire floor waitressing better than any other member of the team. The girls also play music and sing with Lee on Friday and Saturday nights. I cook, waitress, and clean while they fill the room with beautiful music.

Cooking with Kindness

One thing I've known about supporting my body with food is paying attention to the energy that I cook with. This is the most important ingredient—kindness. It takes self-kindness to make the time to learn to cook for our own wellness and kindness to cook for the wellness of a loved one. My dedication to this ingredient has become the roux to all things we do in Pinewood.

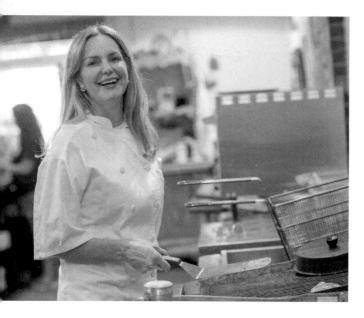

No matter what is going on with me, the moment I enter Pinewood, I shift my energy and open my heart. I always walk behind the line first and check in with my team—each and every one of them—before heading out on the floor to connect to my customers. I need to know that they are okay, and they need to know that I care.

When things get hectic and crazy, I slow the line down and connect with my team and my customers. I remind them all that we cook with real food, and it takes time. The folks who struggle the most are cooks or servers who have worked in kitchens before. The first-timers who cut their teeth in Pinewood only know a kind kitchen, and this helps keep it that way. I have brought many cooks into my kitchen, and they have all struggled with letting go of their workplace anxiety. It's fascinating to me that we eat out more than ever now as a society, but many times we are eating "anxious food."

The point of dining out for most is that it's a treat and thought to be a way to relax from the pressure of home cooking. In Pinewood, people always say how good it feels. This is because we are not just creating an environment for the customers, but for the staff, too. We also pay a living wage, and everyone shares the tips equally—including the cooks, dishwashers, servers, and cashiers. This creates an equal investment in the quality of the food and the service. There is no hierarchy, and this helps avoid martyrs. There are shift leaders, and they guide with kindness.

Creating this has not been easy. It's been downright tough. My body still struggles at times with Hashimoto's fatigue, my rheumatoid arthritis kicks up when I'm stressed or overworked, and if I eat out and I'm "glutened," I miss at least three days of work recovering. Making Pinewood work financially has also been a struggle. It's tough running an organic farm and even tougher running a farm-to-table restaurant. We have to charge more because it takes more hands to pick the bugs off produce

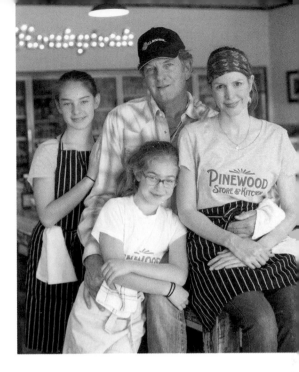

than it does to spray the crops with chemicals. Explaining this to customers is what we do well in Pinewood.

The Future of Pinewood

While all this was going on, I became a contributor on *Today In Nashville,* a morning talk show. It allows me to get off the farm and into city clothes once a week to spread the message of what Pinewood has to offer. I adore the crew and creators of the show, and the opportunity has been so rewarding. Many folks drive from Nashville to eat in Pinewood after seeing my segments, even while some of the diehard Pinewood locals hold firm to the belief that organic is weird food that tastes bad. (Turns out, you can't give everyone what they want.) Since many people were driving so far, I wanted to give them an actual destination, so I took the old abandoned fire hall across the street and turned it into mercantile that sells everything from pickles and jams to saddles and soaps, to blankets, bacon, and eggs. Since we own two buildings, it's technically a downtown! So we put up a sign: WELCOME TO DOWNTOWN PINEWOOD.

In all honesty, though, I was physically and financially worn out running Pinewood, and I needed to take better care of myself and my family. I knew that something needed to shift. Then, in December 2018, a corporation approached me to buy Pinewood Kitchen & Mercantile. Although they had plans to turn it into something other than a restaurant, I have to admit I was tempted. They asked what I wanted for it and matched my price. I called our local realtor and told him about the opportunity to sell.

"No way—you can't!" Dan said. "Do you see how many people have moved to Pinewood in the last three years? They are moving here, yes, because it's beautiful, but also because Pinewood Kitchen gives them a sense of community and fantastic food. Pinewood matters to many."

Without making any firm decisions, we traveled to Florida to see Lee's family for the holidays. Still, I privately mourned the end of Pinewood Kitchen. I cared about my team and the community we had created together, but I knew that alone I was drowning. Aside from the cavalry coming to my rescue, I couldn't see keeping things afloat.

When we returned home, Dan called to say that he'd set up a meeting with a few of the new landowners in Pinewood. They'd each bought farms and weekend homes and loved "the Kitchen." The night before the meeting, I prayed and asked: "If my service is over in Pinewood, I understand. Please lead me to my next purposeful adventure."

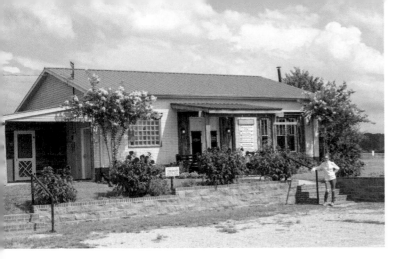

The next day, Lee and I met with the landowners to discuss the future of Pinewood. I took the meeting with no expectations. I was incredibly honest about what Pinewood took to run and keep in business. At the end of the meeting, they were in, and I was in shock. I went home and wept. The cavalry had come to my rescue after all! Our intentions matched, and we were in alignment with maintaining the integrity of Pinewood. In April 2019, we formed a new company, Pinewood Eats. Our goal is to continue to inspire others to connect to real food, ancestral farming, and the investment in rural America. I was no longer alone. I didn't have investors—I had partners as well as an extended Pinewood family: Jamie, Ryan, Adam, and Dierks, along with their wives and children. Pinewood truly is a family affair!

My partners and I recently met with builders to expand our garden house and create an events and education center on the farm. The pressure is off me, and now I roll into Pinewood Kitchen with an even lighter step. My intention is to continue to build with love and kindness and share my knowledge of food and the science behind what we eat so that we can all create our own healing food. That's what the rest of this book aims to do. And, by the way, Pinewood welcomes you to stop by. I'll be there to greet you with open arms and amazing food.

P.S. Remember how I said I wanted to follow in Loretta Lynn's footsteps? Well, her ranch is just a few miles down the road from Pinewood. I made it!

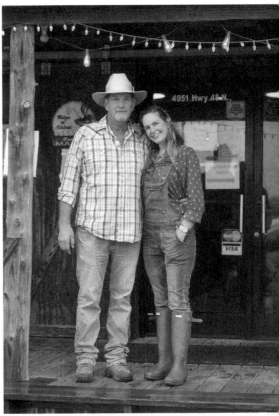

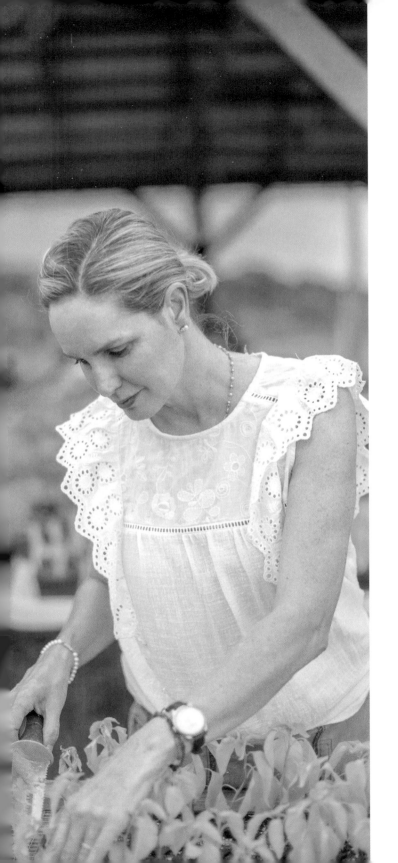

Part Two

The Science: Get to Know Your Gut... So You Can Trust It

I gotta break it to you: We are not alone in these bodies of ours. We share them with trillions of bacteria—on our skin, inside our bodies, and, of course, in our intestines. The colony of intestinal bacteria is called the microbiome. It's an ultra-complex biological system that serves as a lifeline to our cells and organs and influences our health in many ways.

One of its main roles is to create short-chain fatty acids (SCFAs) by processing the fiber from plant foods we eat. These plant-fiber foods are also known as prebiotics. These prebiotics are food for the probiotics, which are the helpful bacteria that support our bodies by countering inflammation and supporting our organs and cells. I refer to these helpful bacteria as "the gut homies," as they are our ride-or-die life partners. If we don't feed them properly, they will die, and unhealthy bacteria will multiply, leading to high levels of inflammation and illness.

Bacteria from Way Back

Tracing where the gut homies came from can go back as far as 300,000 years ago when our ancestors were mainly hunter-gatherers who ate what they could forage: predominantly plant foods, grains, nuts, legumes, and fruits and veggies, all of which contained high amounts of fiber—prebiotic food that nourished our ancient gut homies (aka microbes).

The soil was loaded with even more prebiotic and probiotic bacteria than our current soil, which has been depleted due to overfarming. Each bite our ancestors took of vegetation added prebiotic and probiotic bacteria to their microbiomes. However, as times changed and the agricultural revolution occurred, our ancestors turned away from strictly hunting and gathering and toward cultivated foods, though the basis of their diet was still heavily geared around plants. Sadly, in the 1950s, we moved even further away from our hunting-and-gathering diets and into the industrialized food movement—now known as processed food. This caused the healthy gut microbes to slowly die off because they weren't being replenished and allowed the bad ones to proliferate, causing an imbalance in our guts and a lack of diversity in the microbiome.

For many centuries, we knew very little about bacteria. But once scientists discovered that "germs were the cause of disease," they began to develop various processes of sterilization, which thankfully have saved countless lives. However, the idea that we needed to kill all bacteria was born. Didn't anyone listen to Russian zoologist Èlie Metchnikoff when, in 1907, he suggested that not all bacteria was bad?

During the cholera epidemic of 1892 in France, Metchnikoff mixed bacteria together in a petri dish. Some bacteria stimulated cholera growth while other bacteria hindered it—a finding that took the scientist by surprise. He was also curious why some people lived to be well over 100 years old despite poor hygienic environments. In particular, he discovered a tribe of people living in the Caucasus Mountains who drank fermented yogurt containing the bacteria *Lactobacillus bulgaricus*—what we now identify as a healthy anti-inflammatory bacteria found in fermented kefirs and yogurts. Despite Metchnikoff's assertion, we still saw the rise of disinfectants, sanitizers, and antibiotic cleansers, which do away with the good and the bad bacteria alike.[1]

Fast-forward to today, when the microbiome is recognized as one of the most exciting frontiers in medical research. In the year 2000, when I was becoming very sick with a serious digestive disease (some doctors thought it was Crohn's disease, and another thought it was intestinal cancer), there were only 74 articles published on the microbiome. In 2017, more than 9,600 research articles emerged. Today, that number has quadrupled and is growing each day. So far, we know that there are more than 1,000 gut bacteria species—some are good and others are linked to illness and inflammation.

While some people have problems with certain bacteria, others have no issues; therefore, labeling certain bacteria as inherently bad causes confusion. However, one thing is for sure: We all experience disrupted health when our gut bacteria is out of balance. In 2008, the National Institute of Health launched the Human Microbiome Project, studying 242 individuals and publishing a game-changer paper in 2012 in the scientific journal *Nature*.[2] They found that no one has the same microbiome and that a diverse microbiome was linked to wellness and better health. Folks with a limited community of bacteria had increased health issues from autoimmune diseases, obesity, and cancer.

Unfortunately, in our modern world—as we continue to supersize, sterilize, and stress ourselves out 24/7—it's getting harder to support a diverse microbiome. Many of the foods we eat are depleted of nutrients, many foods contain pesticides and genetically modified ingredients that our bodies cannot process, and our stress levels are sky high. What's more, many people eliminate certain food groups by adhering to certain fad diets. By eliminating entire food groups, we eliminate specific types of healthy gut bacteria for prolonged periods of time, which damages our bodies in the long term. In fact, in a four-generational family study of the microbiome, researchers found that the microbiomes of great grandchildren were missing healthy gut bacteria completely in comparison to their great grandparents![3] Scientists are working to figure out how we can replace these lost bacteria, because, as of now, some cannot be replaced.

So whether it's our environments, our modern lifestyles, or our genes, many things conspire to make our digestive systems work harder. To counter these influences, we need to feed our guts a healthy balance of diverse gut bacteria in the form of probiotic and prebiotic foods.

Building a Better Microbiome

By increasing the amount of probiotic and prebiotic foods you eat, you will do your body good. Prebiotics and probiotics feed your gut homies. As mentioned, these gut homies then create short-chain fatty acids (SCFAs), which are essential for helping to keep your body functioning optimally. For one thing, SCFAs protect the lining of your gut. A weakened gut lining is linked to many health issues, and when the gut lining is weak, inflammation sets in all over the body and in the intestines. When the lining of the intestines is swollen and inflamed, the intestines don't work properly; nothing can be absorbed, and those essential SCFAs can't be created.

SCFAs also help metabolize glucose (sugars) and lipids (fats). By not absorbing fat, we actually gain weight. I know it sounds backward, but it's not: If fat isn't absorbed, the body can't process it. So it hangs out on the side—usually of our jeans! Not absorbing fats means our brains are foggy, our energy levels are low, and our hormones are jacked up. But by supporting the gut microbiome and shifting our gut culture, we can get back to our spry, energetic, quick-witted selves and lose weight and the bloat.

SCFAs also keep our immune system in check, support stem cells, and guide angiogenesis (the body's process of creating new blood vessels). These blood vessels deliver oxygen and nutrients to our body's tissues. This is how we heal wounds and promote new tissue growth. However, angiogenesis also plays a huge role in the formation of cancerous tumors, since tumors need a blood supply to thrive and grow. When the body's angiogenesis system is disrupted, these blood vessels attach to tiny microscopic cancer cells, and—boom—tumors are created. Different health issues occur when this system isn't functioning properly; for example, rheumatoid arthritis is triggered when too much blood flow goes to the joints, and alopecia (hair loss) and diabetes are symptoms of limited blood flow.

SCFAs are the muscle behind stem cells and our body's ability to create new ones. Three of the most powerful SCFAs are butyrate, propionate, and acetate, and each participate in unique ways within the body. Propionate can lower cholesterol, reduce inflammation, and protect against plaque in the arteries. It also helps improve digestion and activate immune cells. Butyrate is key to a healthy colon by serving as energy that fuels healthy colon cells and playing a big role in fighting inflammation all over the body. It helps wound healing by stimulating angiogenesis. The real whopper is that butyrate guides stem cells to regenerate damaged organ cells. SCFAs are linked to fighting obesity because acetate is released into peripheral tissues where it stimulates the hormone leptin, which suppresses hunger and leads to weight loss.

The Link Between Gut Bacteria and Anxiety & Depression

Our gut homies don't just help with our physical health issues, but with our emotional health, too. The bacteria *Bifidobacterium* has been shown to reduce stress and anxiety through a unique gut-brain interaction. Researchers at the Netherlands Organization for Applied Scientific Research designed a study to test whether eating chocolate—a prebiotic food—could mitigate stress-related effects on the microbiome. They studied thirty healthy folks between the ages of eighteen and thirty-five. They first established their self-reported stress levels via a survey and then divided them into high-anxiety and low-anxiety groups, testing the blood and urine of both groups for stress markers at the start. Then the participants received 40 grams of dark chocolate with 74% cocoa—the equivalent of a commercially available medium-size dark chocolate bar—every day for two weeks.

The researchers found that when the participants ate dark chocolate for two weeks, their levels of stress markers (cortisol and adrenaline) decreased in their urine as well as two markers called p-cresol and hippurate, which are metabolites of good gut bacteria. Eating high levels of pure dark chocolate reduced anxiety levels in high-anxiety folks down to the levels of low-anxiety folks. You know why? Because cacao—the plant that dark chocolate comes from—is a prebiotic food for the good gut bacteria. Milk chocolate, on the other hand, will only jack up the gut with an excess of sugar and dairy and not enough cacao, the prebiotic fiber needed to shift the gut microbiome.[4]

The balance of gut homies has also been linked to lowered rates of depression, which by the way, is the second leading cause of disability in the United States. The drugs used to treat depression are selective serotonin reuptake inhibitors such as Prozac, Paxil, and Celexa. They boost the activity of the serotonin-signaling system, which psychiatry had long thought is exclusively located in the brain. But now we know that 95 percent of the body's serotonin is actually contained in specialized cells *in the gut!*

These serotonin-containing cells are influenced by what we eat and by the prebiotic fibers we feed *or don't feed* the good gut homies. When the gut bacteria are rolling at full speed and supported, they release certain kinds of gut microbes that communicate via the signals the brain sends regarding our emotional state. These brain-communicating cells are tightly connected to sensory nerves, which signal directly back into the brain's emotional-regulating centers, making them an important hub within the gut-brain axis.

This hub is where we find the connection between microbes and their metabolites and how they play an important and largely understudied role in the development of depression. I love that science is digging deep because we know that depression can be hereditary, but now we are learning exactly how it's passed down generationally through the gut microbiome of our relatives. (Y'all should know I'm jumping outta my seat cheering as I write this. Because if we can get in our kitchens and use food as a way to help us find emotional balance, we gain back our confidence and our ability to create joyful, incredible lives.)

I have slipped into dark places in my life. The death of my momma and friends in two separate car accidents, all the moves we've made as a family, the struggles and stress of running a farm, ranch, and restaurant, and the disappointments of normal life, plus the major imbalance of gut microbes has caused me to hit the emotional concrete a few too many times. Finding my way back up has been a journey of its own, and I have seen a huge positive change in my emotional self since healing my gut.

Share and Share Alike

Did you know that families or folks who cohabitate together have similar microbiomes? It makes sense that our bacteria are all over the place—on our skin, scalps, drinking cups, toilet seats, showers, and eating utensils. Now we are discovering that families have similar weight issues not just because they share the same diets, but because they share similar microbes. Our microbiomes can shift depending on who we live with (wow, right?). We even share similar microbiomes as our pets and vice versa![5]

Rotate Your Plate:
The Power of a Diverse Gut

When folks ask me to help them learn to cook healthy, I first tell them to spend a few days paying attention to what they eat the most often. Once we do this, we can identify our excess. Some folks are dry, crunchy snack eaters—and these snacks can be wheat free, corn free, or gluten free. But what dry, crunchy processed snacks do, even if they are organic, is absorb water from the intestines. Compare this to soaking a piece of bread in a dish of water—most of the water will disappear as the bread absorbs it. That's what happens in our intestines. Plus, if we grab a dry, crunchy snack, we aren't grabbing foods that contain plant fiber, or prebiotics, which are good for our guts.

Our excesses vary. Some folks can't get enough cheese each day; some chow down on meat as the focus of their plate; and yes, eating the same veggies too much creates an excess, too. Sugar is a sneaky one. It's a nibble here and there that wreaks havoc on our guts. An excess of something means we are limiting our diet and the microbiome, and therefore, we are not feeding the good gut homies what they need. That's how we create a real imbalance—we don't eat enough variety.

How We Do It in Pinewood

Because Pinewood Farms is a biodynamic farm, our gardens are created with the biodiversity of a natural ecosystem. We are mindful of planting a variety of herbs, flowers, berries, fruits, nuts, and grains, and having open pastures, orchards, mushrooms, native plants, and pollinators, such as bees. All of this supports the giant organism of our farm. This organism feeds us and our community's microbiome as we serve these foods in our Pinewood Kitchen.

We apply this same mind-set with our livestock. We move our cattle three times a day in the high-grass season to keep them balanced in their

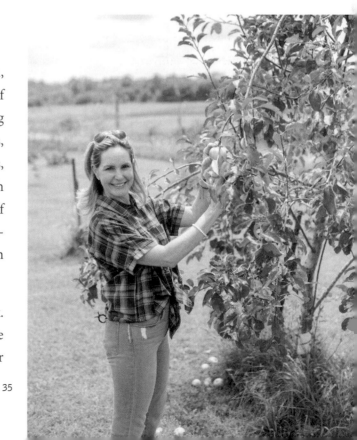

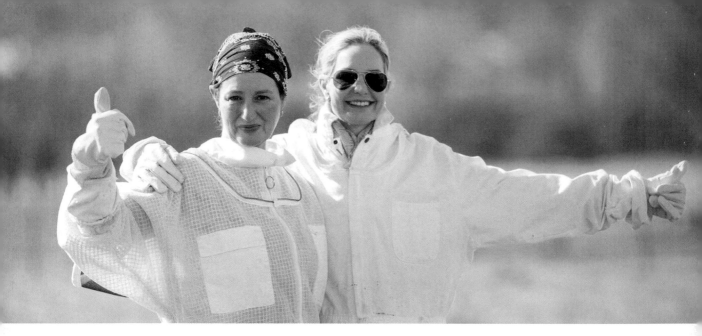

wellness. Moving them from pasture to pasture each day helps because each pasture has a different nutritional profile depending on what type of grass is planted there and how much sunlight and water it gets.

We also rotate our crops each season and allow our soil time to recover. During the recovery time, we feed the microbiome of the soil by planting different types of cover crops while it rests, which creates a diverse microbe culture in our compost (aka natural fertilizer). This ultimately keeps the integrity of the soil intact so that the food we grow is loaded with nutrients. Eating a rotational, seasonal diet is how I keep my own microbiome and those who dine in Pinewood in balance. We serve what we grow and create the menu so that it matches the rotation of crops coming off the farm.

Stocking a Probiotic Pantry: Fermented Foods Are Your Gut's Best Friend

Feeding the good gut bacteria isn't as complicated as you would think. You can improve your gut biome by eating fermented foods like sauerkraut, kimchi, miso paste, koji rice, and homemade yogurt from goat milk, coconut milk, or other vegan milks. You don't have to make your own; there are plenty of store-bought versions to choose from. Just be sure to read ingredients and avoid products that are high in sugar.

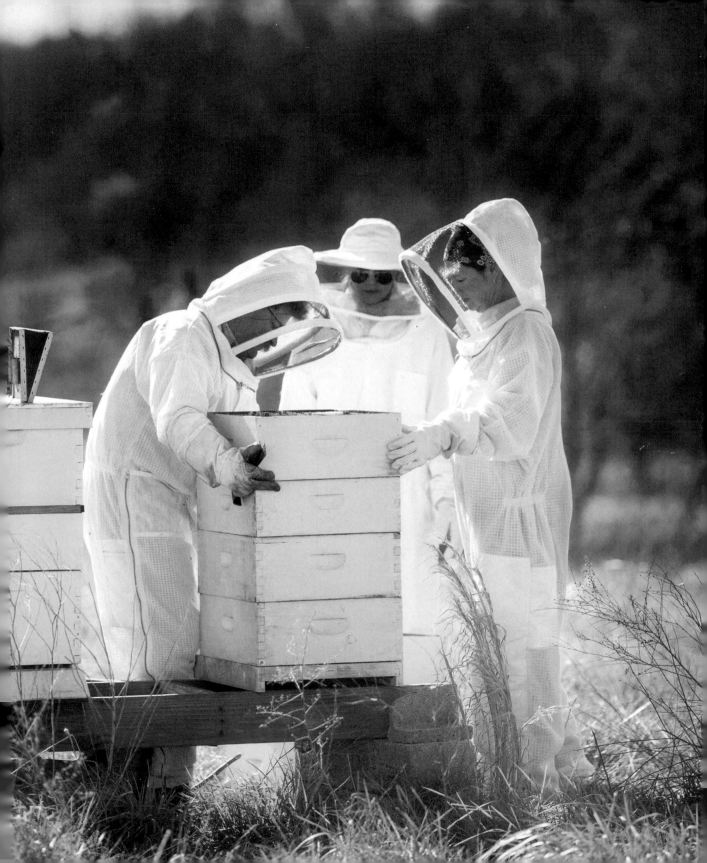

The Good, the Bad, and the Ugly: Know the Gut Homies

As I mentioned earlier, we know that there are more than 1,000 gut bacteria species. They aren't all bad or all good (whether they're ugly or not is up to you to decide). I've handpicked a few of the more common ones along with some interesting tidbits of information just to give you an idea of who's living in your gut and to what effect.

Actinobacteria is considered beneficial, along with its phylum (meaning the smaller levels of bacteria located within a bacteria, or, as I think of them, as the major gut homies' posse). These are commonly found in probiotic supplements.

Bacteroidetes is a neutral bacteria and is found in folks with higher protein and animal fat consumption. If it should grow to excess, it increases inflammation. High levels of this bacteria are found in people who have been on the keto diet (high in fats, low in carbs with adequate protein) long term. Bacteroidetes make up the second-largest culture of the microbiome. Many of them are SCFA-producing bacteria. We like those!

Bifidobacteria and its phylum **Actinobacteria** is totally beneficial and commonly included in probiotic supplements.

Firmicutes make up the majority of the microbiome, and they are the most diverse. The most beneficial SCFAs-producing bacteria are within the firmicutes phylum, but other strains of them have been shown to be pathogenic, meaning they can be harmful and make us sick.

Lactobacillus casei and its phylum **Firmicutes** is found in fermented dairy products. This is beneficial and is usually included in probiotic supplements. Studies show that it is protective against gastroenteritis, diabetes, cancer, obesity, and even postpartum depression. That's a gut homie that's gotch ya back.[6]

Proteobacteria is considered harmful in excess. Studies have found an increased amount of this bacteria in metabolic disorders and in people with inflammatory bowel disease (IBD).[7]

Verrucomicrobia is a small culture of bacteria and newly discovered phylum. Within verrucomicrobia is where we find *Akkermansia,* a bacteria located in the mucosal lining of the intestines. It is a tiny colony but does a big job by keeping inflammation at bay in the lining of the intestines. *Akkermansia* combats obesity, improves blood glucose metabolism, and improves the efficacy of certain cancer treatments. That's a supa-dupa gut homie!

I make my own vegan yogurts from nuts, and if your digestive system can handle cow's dairy yogurts, then go for it. In addition, all kinds of fermented veggies and fruits can be helpful for gut health. In Pinewood Kitchen, we pickle everything we can to preserve it. When I was healing my gut, I added probiotics to my diet in the form of fermented foods. This is part of how I healed the large ulceration in my intestines. The scientific jury is still out on whether pharmaceutical probiotics work for all folks. That's because each person has a specific microbiome. In the future, as we personalize medicine, we will start with the mapping of our individual biomes, and it will become clearer as to which probiotic supplements to take.

If you have any questions about what's right for your gut, seek out a functional medicine specialist. He or she can help you make the best choices. (If you have or suspect you have histamine intolerance, turn to page 52.) But if you know fermented foods are friendly, put the following on your grocery list.

Sauerkraut

Sauerkraut originated in China through trade routes and early merchants brought it to Eastern and Western European cuisine. It's been a part of a Chinese medicine healing diet for centuries and now we understand why. A one-cup serving can contain up to 5 trillion lactobacilli bacteria. This particular bacteria is what's found in most traditional probiotics because it's linked to lowering inflammation and supporting intestinal stem cells.[8] Shredded fermented cabbage (aka sauerkraut) also releases bioactive compounds (that is, they have a biological effect) with antiangiogenic properties, meaning they slow the blood supply to tumors and they can kill cancer cells directly.[9]

Kimchi

Kimchi is a dang showstopper. In Korean, it comes from the word "gimchi," which means "submerged vegetables." It's made from chili peppers, garlic, ginger, scallions, radishes, cabbage, and a fermented seafood product called jeotgal. You can find it in almost any market. It's usually served as a side dish, and I love it with eggs, on tacos, or just a scoop of it by itself.

It's pretty much the king of probiotic foods as it delivers loads of bioactives to our gut. Many of the bacteria found in kimchi are the same as the ones located in our own microbiomes: Bacteroidetes, Firmicutes, and *Lactobacillus*, among many others. The scientists at the World Institute of Kimchi in Korea (Yep, there is such a place!) discovered a new bacteria called *Lactobacillus kimchii* that produces K2, or menaquinone. This is an antiangiogenic bioactive that's also found in dark meat chicken. (If you need a reminder, antiangiogenic bioactives can help halt the formation of blood vessels to a tumor.)

Another bacterial compound also found in kimchi is propionic acid, an SCFA that lowers cholesterol, reduces inflammation, prevents buildup of plaque in arteries, and improves digestive health. In addition, the *Lactobacillus plantarum* growing in kimchi is also protective against influenza A. But the *insanely* cool news is that extracts from kimchi have been found to kill cancer cells from the colon, bone, and liver, as well as leukemia![10] You can purchase sauerkraut and kimchi in almost any grocery store. Bubbies Pickles and Bubbies Sauerkraut is right alongside the kimchi in my local market.

More Gut Game-Changers

Now that you have fermented foods on your shopping list, get ready to add some other gut-friendly foods to your list so that you can work these into your weekly rotation. You'll see most of these included in the ingredients of some of the recipes in Part Three.

Walnuts

According to a study at The University of Munich, folks who ate twenty-one walnut halves a day for three weeks increased their SCFAs for butyrate, propionate, and acetate. (Don't remember what these are or what they do? That's okay; see page 32.)[11]

Beans

Beans are super good for your gut health, but they can be tough to digest because most of us don't have enough of the good gut homies that break them down. To help with digestion, you need to soak dried beans overnight and remove the foam, and then rinse them well. (You'll learn all about the "Rules of Beans" in Part Three.) In some cases, canned beans are fine, but you gotta buy organic (check out the Eden Foods brand) and rinse them really well.

I know from firsthand experience that working legumes (beans, peas, and lentils) into your diet can be tricky, especially if you don't have the bacteria in place to break them down. I started off with small portions of beans (less than a quarter cup at a time, maybe twice a week), or I pureed them. I make a black bean soup that is pureed and therefore easier to digest.

If you avoid beans completely, you are starving out the gut bacteria that feed off of them. Scientists at the University of Guelph in Ontario, Canada, studied the effects of two kinds of beans—navy and black beans—on the microbiome. They found that both kinds of beans supported the healthy bacteria that create all three of the SCFAs, and they increased *Ruminococcus* bacteria, which break down plant cells (another way to create SCFAs). Researchers uncovered the effect beans have on the mucosal lining of the intestines, as well as gut barrier function, both of which are linked to gut bacteria. We need this mucosal lining; the stronger it is, the healthier we are, since it prevents substances that can leak from the gut (see "What Is Leaky Gut?" below).[12]

In a recent study involving mice, researchers found that beans improved the intestinal lining. They found that the protective mucus-secreting cells of the upper colon increased by 60 percent in mice fed navy beans, and by 120 percent in the mice fed black beans. In the lower colon, mucus cells increased by 57 percent with black bean chow.[13] Chickpeas, lentils, and peas are in the legume family along with beans, and they influence the gut in the same way.

What Is Leaky Gut?

When we don't have a balance of good gut bacteria as a result of diet, medications, or illness, we become susceptible to a weakened lining of the intestines, which can result in "leaky gut." When the tight junctions that control what the intestines can absorb don't work properly, it allows larger (but still tiny) substances to cross over into the bloodstream where they don't belong. (This is called permeability.)

Folks with Crohn's disease, celiac disease, those having undergone chemotherapy, and those who consume large amounts of aspirin and alcohol tend to have higher rates of "leaky gut." Research is now being done to see if leaky gut is linked to many autoimmune diseases, heart disease, cancer, asthma, and eczema. Stay tuned for more on this in the future, and in the meantime, try making the right choices to keep your gut happy.

Olive Oil

Humans have been using olive oil for 4,000 years. Most of the olive oil Americans consume comes from Spain, Italy, Greece, and Morocco, and the olives they grow contain high levels of bioactive polyphenols (supportive micronutrients from plants). Extra-virgin olive oil is made from fresh pressed olives, and it contains the highest levels of bioactives and the best flavor. All these polyphenols are why olive oil is antiangiogenic, anti-inflammatory, and antioxidant, and helps defend our bodies from cancer.

Olives and fresh-pressed olive oil are some of the best foods to support a healthy gut microbiome. Olives grown in arid areas require less care, as there are fewer bugs, molds, and fungi; therefore, there are fewer pesticides used on non-organic olives grown in arid places. Fewer pesticides are also good for the gut microbiome.

Olive oil is one of the only fats that has been proven in a lab to decrease the risks of cancer. A study conducted by the Istituto di Ricerche Farmacologiche Mario Negri and the University of Milan examined 27,000 subjects in Italy for their consumption of extra-virgin olive oil, butter, margarine, and seed oil. They discovered that 3 to 4 tablespoons per day of olive oil was associated with a reduced risk of esophageal cancer by 70 percent, laryngeal cancer by 60 percent, oral and pharyngeal cancer by 60 percent, ovarian cancer by 32 percent, and colorectal cancer by 17 percent! They did not see any of these benefits with seed oils, and more important, butter was associated with an increased risk of esophageal, oral, and pharyngeal cancer by twofold![14] Dang it, pass the olive oil!

Fraudulent Olive Oil?

It's been reported that 80% of the olive oil on the market is fraudulent. In other words, it doesn't actually contain olives.[15] After a lot of press exposure, one company stepped up to offer 100% transparency: Pompeian Olive Oil. The owners, David and Galit, have since become my friends. Under David's leadership, Pompeian has created an FDA-monitoring system to guarantee that the olive oil they sell is 100% true olive oil.

David's passion for transparency in the real-food movement matches my desire to inspire people to eat wholesome food. David and Galit invited me to join them on a press tour to Morocco to visit their olive oil farms, which was a trip I will never forget. The food, the people, and the rich history of the country inspired me to create the recipe for Chickpea Cauliflower "Couscous" (page 193).

Mushrooms

Mushrooms are adaptogens, a naturally occurring substance that protects the body from stress by stabilizing and optimizing its physiological functions. Adaptogens boost immunity, protect us from disease, and promote overall health and wellness. Many plants and mushrooms, such as ginseng root, holy basil, cordyceps, and reishi are well known for their adaptogenic properties. What's super cool about these adaptogenic mushrooms is that, true to their name, they *adapt* their healing abilities to whatever your body specifically needs at any given time to restore you to peak functionality. Aside from cordyceps, you can find these mushrooms dried and/or fresh and use them in dishes, make teas with them, or take them as supplements. (Cordyceps is only available in supplement form.)

Reishi

Reishi, also known in Chinese medicine as *lingzhi*, is considered the queen of mushrooms. Reishi is a revitalizer and was reserved for emperors and other royalty in ancient China. Reishi has been used in Chinese medicine for more than 2,000 years. Its adaptogenic properties help stabilize our immune system so that it operates at its full potential, protecting us from pathogens like viruses, bacteria, and parasites.

Reishi polysaccharides (a form of carbohydrates in the mushroom) have been shown to lower blood pressure, stabilize blood sugar, lower cholesterol, and inhibit tumor growth in some cancers. Reishi even helps us reach hormonal balance by supporting the endocrine system. In my life, reishi mushrooms have supported me by helping fight gut inflammation; they can alter the ratio of unhealthy bacteria and support the good bacteria. Reishi mushrooms have been shown to help in digesting a high-fat diet, so if you are rockin' that keto diet, add some high-quality reishi powder to your smoothie, coffee, or tea.[16]

Chaga

Chaga is the king of mushrooms and is known to ward off common cold viruses, support hair and skin, and lower inflammation caused by high stress. This mushroom dates back to seventeenth-century Russia, where it was used for everything—from digestive distress to cancer. Dual-extracted chaga is one of the most potent sources of antioxidants in the world. One cup of chaga tea packs the same number of antioxidants as thirty pounds of carrots, and y'all know antioxidants protect our bodies from free radicals. It's said that Tsar Vladimir Monomakh, who ruled the twelfth-century Kievan Rus', used chaga to cure his lip cancer. That's because chaga has the ability to boost the production of lymphocytes, a type of white blood cell that regulates the immune response to infectious microorganisms.[17]

Cordyceps (Supplements)

Cordyceps are known to increase energy and reduce fatigue. Having Hashimoto's disease (an autoimmune disease that attacks the thyroid) means I have gone toe to toe with fatigue and brain fog. Adding cordyceps into my diet has helped me stay in the game of my insanely full life. I take three capsules a day. They have been a centerpiece of traditional Chinese medicine for more than 1,300 years. Cordyceps are anti-inflammatory, they help with our blood flow, support heart health, and lower cholesterol. Plus, they contain a chemical compound called cordycepic acid, which is known to shrink tumors and stimulate lymphocyte production, helping to kill harmful foreign bodies in the immune system.[18]

Lion's Mane

Lion's mane is a digestive-healing mushroom. I wish I'd known about this mushroom twelve years ago. I wish I could tell every single person who suffers from digestive distress and inflammation to try it out. I personally take three capsules a day. It's known for its culinary goodness, and it's used in traditional Chinese medicine to help those suffering from digestive distress and digestive cancers. It's also anti-inflammatory, antibacterial, and immunomodulating (which means it helps support and balance the immune system).

Lion's mane mushroom was studied in the lab at Jiangnan University in China to test its effects on the microbiome. They fed mice with severe gut inflammation the human equivalent of one tablespoon of lion's mane mushroom. The results showed that lion's mane could decrease the symptoms and proteins associated with gut inflammation by as much as 40 percent. The mushroom also increased the healthy bacteria *Akkermansia* while decreasing the harmful sulfur toxin–producing *Desulfovibrio*. As someone with inflammatory bowel issues, lion's mane is my homie.[19]

Cutting-edge studies about lion's mane show its neurological effects on the brain. It has the ability to repair and regenerate neurons in your body, resulting in an overall increased cognitive function. Lion's mane also has been known to reduce the effects of neurological diseases like Parkinson's disease, Alzheimer's disease, and dementia.[20]

Taking capsules and tinctures of lion's mane is something everyone can do with ease, and cooking lion's mane mushroom is crazy simple, too—just chop and sauté in olive oil or ghee.

Shiitake

We grow plenty of shiitake on the farm; actually, I think of it as *raising* shiitake because mushrooms are living beings. Do you know how long it takes to raise a shiitake mushroom on a farm? Six to nine months! We start by drilling holes into logs and placing wet mushroom spores into the logs. Then we gather them up and drive the logs out to a shady spot. We stand them up in a shiitake mushroom circle, and there they sit for months until they are ready to harvest. Then, it's shiitake party time. We drive out with anticipation and then we carefully cut the mushrooms off the logs.

The use of shiitake dates back to 100 CE in China when they were commonly used to treat upper-respiratory illness, to increase energy and decrease fatigue, and promote circulation. Today we know they are such a powerhouse food because they contain seven of the nine essential amino acids (the proteins that must be consumed from outside of the body as we do not create them). They have been wonderful for me, as they also contain a slew of digestive enzymes and vitamins D and B. They also help the body stimulate white blood cells that help us fight infections. Shiitake mushrooms support the liver, which, in turn, makes our skin shine bright, since our skin is a direct reflection of how well our liver is functioning. They are helpful to the heart and to the microbiome by supporting vascular health and lowering cholesterol.

I put shiitake mushrooms in everything from soups, omelets, and simple sautés to slow-cooked meats. If you can't find them fresh, order them dried online.

Maitake

In Japanese *maitake* means "dancing mushroom." This is appropriate for me, considering my Pine-wood Kitchen has a lot of dancing going on inside.

Maitake has super immunomodulating abilities, and where it shines is its SX-fraction, a water-soluble compound so named because of its ability to counteract the effects of Syndrome X. This is a metabolic syndrome, not a disease, that involves high cholesterol, high blood pressure, and excess fat. Because of the maitake's SX-fraction, it can help reduce blood glucose levels, blood pressure, and excess weight, which is a game-changer in fighting obesity and the onset of diabetes. But because it's an adaptogen, it helps everyone who takes it. Maitake also contains D-fraction, which has been studied to prevent breast cancer—another reason to get your maitake dancing on![21]

I sauté it and add it to soups, stews, and veggies. It's got a great flavor and is said to be one of the umamis of cooking. "Umami" means *pleasant, savory taste* in Japanese; it's one of the five basic tastes.

White Button Mushrooms

Don't forget these common fun guys! They, too, are loaded with vitamin D and they are immuno-modulators, which aid in supporting and balancing the immune system. The department of plant pathology at Penn State released a report stating that button mushrooms have been found to be effective at treating breast, colon, and prostate cancer.[22]

Researchers at the Beckman Research Institute tested thirty-six men with prostate cancer. They started these men out with 8 grams of white button mushroom extract and increased it to 14 grams per day for three months. By the end of the three months, over one-third of the men had experienced reductions in PSA levels, indicating improvement. Some of the men experienced what the researchers call a complete response after their PSA levels went down so far that they were undetectable. The PSA levels remained this way for the following thirty months.[23]

Researchers at Penn State also studied the influence of eating white button mushrooms on the microbiome of mice and found the increase of healthy gut bacteria, *Akkermansia* and Bacteroide-tes, which are supporters of the gut lining. Also, Firmicutes phylum, a harmful species of bacteria, decreased.[24]

Prebiotic & Probiotic Powerhouses

In addition to all of the gut-friendly foods I've already mentioned, there's a host more. I try to work all of the following prebiotic foods into my diet weekly. We grow a lot of these in Pinewood, but you don't need to be a farmer to harvest these goodies. Shop your local grocery store for fresh produce or, if unavailable, buy frozen or dried without preservatives.

- Apricots
- Arugula
- Asparagus
- Black tea (organic)
- Broccoli and broccoli leaves
- Cabbage
- Cauliflower
- Cherries
- Chickpeas
- Cranberries

- Dark chocolate (containing at least 74% cacao)
- Kale
- Kiwi*
- Lentils
- Sweet potato
- Pomegranate juice
- Organic Cabernet Franc**
- Root veggies (rutabagas, turnips, and parsnips)
- Pumpkins and pumpkinseeds

The National University of Singapore conducted a study to examine the effect of kiwi fruit on the gut microbiome. They fed six women the equivalent of two kiwi fruits a day for four days (a total of eight kiwis) and studied the effects in their fecal matter. The changes were rapid: lactobacillus was increased by 35 percent within 24 hours of eating kiwi. Bifidobacteria increased gradually by 17 percent over four days. Both of these gut homies are major creators of SCFAs that help keep the gut lining in perfect condition.[25]

** *Organic Cabernet Franc is red wine made from the Cabernet grape that the gut homies love—just don't overdo it because too much alcohol will throw the gut off. Doctors say to consume no more than one 5-ounce glass of wine per day or you will negate any health effects.[26]*

Incorporating these powerhouses into your diet is a way to dip your toes in the prebiotic food world with some of the most potent available sources.

Berry Good for You

Most mornings I start my day with a smoothie, so you'll find a few of my favorite smoothie recipes in the breakfast section of Part Three. I load up my smoothies with gut-healthy fruits and berries because it's an easy way to get the good stuff in while allowing my intestines to take it easy digesting. You don't have to blend 'em, though; these gut-friendly ingredients can make great toppings for salads and in main dishes and desserts. Here's a list of the fruit and berries I use in my rotation and why:

- **Seasonal berries.** This includes strawberries, blueberries, raspberries, blackberries, and cranberries. Their strong colors are outward signs of their potent bioactives and antioxidants. They are low in sugar, and the gut homies love them. In a big old study done by the European Prospective Investigation into cancer and nutrition, the diet and health patterns of 478,535 people across ten European countries were examined over two decades for their association with cancer and other chronic diseases, including cardiovascular disease. The most important conclusion was that berry consumption was linked to lower risks of cancer. People who ate one-fifth cup of berries of any type per day were found to have a 22 percent reduced risk of developing lung cancer.[27]

- **Black raspberry.** Black raspberry was shown to be super supportive for people with Barrett's esophagus, a type of precancerous lesion. The black raspberries made the lesions less aggressive, reducing the cellular changes that lead to cancer. Black raspberries also have the same effect on precancerous colon polyps. Having had major intestinal issues and digestive issues for most of my life, my colon health is everything to me. For this reason, black raspberries find their way into my smoothies regularly. If you can't find actual black raspberries, you can order black raspberry extract and add that to your smoothies.[28]

- **Blueberries.** Another widespread study of 75,929 women showed that those who ate one cup of fresh blueberries per week showed a 31 percent reduced risk for breast cancer.[29] I am sure to add at least ¼ cup of fresh blueberries to my smoothies, making it super easy to get my one cup's worth in a week. Y'all, one cup of blueberries is easy peasy to add into our diets! I buy frozen blueberries when we run out of fresh ones.

- **Cranberries.** Frozen cranberries are one of my favorites to add to a smoothie, as they brighten it up and contain high levels of bioactive proanthocyanidins (the deep red and blue Proanthocyanidins colors in fruits and veggies), which have anticancer and antiangiogenic effects. However, the real deal for me is that cranberries are the most favorite food of *Akkermansia muciniphila*, a gut homie located in the mucosal lining of the small intestines. *Akkermansia* is a small colony of gut bacteria but it's one of the most important because it fights inflammation in the intestines and it's linked to helping combat obesity. It loves whole cranberries because cranberries contain proanthocyanidins that help increase the mucous lining in the gut; in a nutshell, cranberries help support the ecosystem that *Akkermansia* needs to thrive.

- **Mangoes.** I love mangoes for their sweet-tart taste but also because they contain a unique bioactive called mangiferin that has antitumor, antidiabetic, and pro-regenerative properties.

- **Pomegranates.** *Akkermansia* also loves pomegranates so I add ¼ cup of pure pomegranate juice to my smoothies. Researchers at the University of California Los Angeles studied the effects of pure pomegranate juice on the microbiome. People who drank one cup of pure pomegranate juice per day for four weeks increased the presence of *Akkermansia* by 71 percent![30]

- **Stone fruits (such as cherries).** Stone fruits are also loved by *Akkermansia*, and cherries, in particular, help *Akkermansia* strengthen their colony in the colon (keeping inflammation out of the colon is how we begin to prevent colon cancer and colitis). According to the U.S. National Cancer Institute and the University of Illinois at Chicago, consuming two medium-size stone fruits per day is associated with a 66 percent decreased risk of esophageal cancer and an 18 percent decreased risk of lung cancer in men.[31]

- **Sour cherries.** Sour cherries help curb the pain and inflammation associated with rheumatoid arthritis because they contain high levels of an active ingredient called cyanidin with way fewer side effects than an aspirin. Don't forget plums, which actually have three times the amount of cancer-fighting polyphenols compared to peaches, and in a laboratory study, a carotenoid called lutein found in apricots prevented the formation of brain-damaging beta-amyloid fibrils that are linked to abnormal angiogenesis found in Alzheimer's disease.[32]

- **Strawberries.** Strawberries are also loaded with a powerful bioactive known as ellagic acid, one of the major players that helps me keep my rheumatoid arthritis at bay. When you bite into a tart strawberry, remember that it's the tartness of the berry that has antiangiogenic activity. Camarosa strawberries from the Ohio Valley have some of the highest levels of ellagic acid.

Let's Chat About Sugar, Sugar

Sugar is sugar. Whether it's monk sugar, coconut sugar, brown sugar, honey, or maple syrup, none of it is great for the gut, and the jury is still out on stevia, though it seems to have the least negative effect on the gut. I'd love to tell you otherwise. I do my best to avoid sugar, but when I am making something that calls for sugar, I try to lessen the negative punch by using honey from our farm when we have it available, and I use it sparingly because we have a limited supply.

I use coconut sugar, too, because it retains quite a bit of the nutrients found in the coconut palm, such as zinc, iron, calcium, and potassium. Plus, it has polyphenols and antioxidants. The reason it's lower on the glycemic index is because it contains inulin, a prebiotic fiber. Mind you, if you go crazy and coconut-sugar everything, it's not going to help your gut.

Monk fruit sugar is becoming more popular. It comes from a small, green Southeast Asian gourd that looks similar to a melon. It was first used by Buddhist monks in the thirteenth century—hence the name monk fruit. Monk fruit sweeteners are created from the fruit's extracts and can be blended with dextrose or other ingredients. It is 150 to 200 times sweeter than regular sugar. Folks like it because it has zero calories, zero carbs, zero sodium, and no fat.

The Deal with Stevia

Stevia is a sweetener that's often used in place of sugar, and you'll see it as a substitution in some of the ingredient lists in Part Three. When using stevia, make sure you are using a pure source. The dried, ground leaves are best, followed by good-quality extracts; always buy organic to make sure you're getting the purest form available.

Stevia is a bushy shrub that's part of the sunflower family, and it's actually easy to make. You would grow it the same way you might grow basil in the right climate. When it's time to harvest, cut off the branches at the base of the plant. Wash them well and pick the leaves off. Then dry the leaves for at least 12 hours in the sun. Once they are dry, put them in a spice grinder and—boom—you've got stevia!

Stevia is super sweet—200 to 300 times sweeter than table sugar. A little goes a *long* way. Here is a simple conversion chart for swapping out regular sugar for stevia:

Sugar Amount	Equivalent Stevia Powdered Extract	Equivalent Stevia Liquid Concentrate
1 cup	1 teaspoon	1 teaspoon
1 tablespoon	¼ teaspoon	6 to 9 drops
1 teaspoon	A pinch to $\frac{1}{16}$ teaspoon	2 to 4 drops

Food Allergies, Sensitivities, Intolerances to Gluten, & More

As food allergies and intolerances increase, educating ourselves on what this all means and how we can better serve ourselves or loved ones with these intolerances makes life easier and less painful. There are more and more tests appearing that track sensitivity levels to foods, and we are learning through microbiome testing that these sensitivities are linked to an overabundance or an underabundance of particular bacteria. In the meantime, Pinewood Kitchen is busy educating and cooking for all different types of food allergies and sensitivities.

We are unique in Pinewood because we listen to our customers and do our best to educate our staff about all the ingredients in our recipes. Our cooks are trained to create food for individual needs, including the following:

Food Allergies

When certain proteins in food trigger a harmful immune response, an allergic reaction occurs. The proteins that trigger the reaction are called allergens. The symptoms of an allergic reaction to food can range from mild (itchy mouth, a few hives) to severe (throat tightening, difficulty breathing). Digestive reactions can include diarrhea, intestinal spasms, nausea, vomiting, and gas or bloating. Some people react with a stuffy nose, runny nose, or headache. Extreme reactions like anaphylaxis can be sudden and lead to death.

There are more than 170 foods that cause allergic reactions. You can technically be allergic to any food, but the top-eight major food allergens are milk, eggs, peanuts, tree nuts, wheat, soy, fish and crustacean shellfish, and, in the case of alpha-gal syndrome, even meat.[33] But humans can be allergic to anything.

In Pinewood, we are mindful of all these allergies. Before Pinewood Kitchen, I never realized how prevalent the alpha-gal allergy is. Alpha-gal syndrome is a recently identified type of food allergy to red meat although some people are also allergic to pork and lamb. In the United States, the condition most often begins when a Lone Star tick bite transmits a sugar molecule called alpha-gal into the body. In some people, this triggers an immune reaction that later produces mild to severe allergic reactions when they eat red meat. This tick is found predominantly in the Southeastern United States, but these ticks and this allergy are spreading all over the country. Alpha-gal syndrome also has been diagnosed in Europe, Asia, and Australia, where other types of ticks carry the alpha-gal molecule, and Australia has super high numbers of it. The response to the alpha-gal allergy can be severe digestive distress that sends folks to the hospital or causes anaphylaxis. We have plenty of people in Pinewood who carry EpiPens. We handle their food separately and carefully by keeping it as far from beef and pork as possible.

Current statistics estimate that 32 million Americans have food allergies, including 5.6 million children under age 18. That's one in thirteen children, or roughly two in every classroom. About 40 percent of children with food allergies are allergic to more than one food. What's really crazy is that the Centers for Disease Control and Prevention reports that the rate of food allergies in children has increased by 50 percent since 1997. This means there is a multiplier effect here, and these numbers are increasing exponentially. This is the beginning of an epidemic. Culinary training will soon need to include alternative ways of cooking and running a professional kitchen.

Histamine Intolerance

I had never heard of histamine intolerance until my homie Heather (also the photographer who shot the cover photo) was diagnosed at the Cleveland Clinic. She had suffered for years with major fatigue, migraines, and constant connective tissue itching and was originally diagnosed with Hodgkin's lymphoma. She stayed with me for a few weeks to learn to cook and did well for a while eating super-clean, fresh foods. Then she went down hard, landing in the Cleveland Clinic's functional medicine program. They discovered that she is genetically deficient in the enzymes

Put Your Gut to the Test

Gut microbiome tests, which you can take at home, offer a wealth of detailed information. I recently took the Viome Gut Intelligence Test, which shows what bacteria is found in my gut, what microbes I'm lacking, what foods are recommended to shift my gut community, and what foods I need to cut back on because they don't serve my body. As I've mentioned, the gut microbiome can shift with just one meal, but according to Viome, although we may experience improvement in just a few weeks, it is best to retest after ninety days to see if we've made a lasting improvement.

This test is dang encouraging to me. Once we see that we can help ourselves feel better, a big plate of inspiration is served, and the desire to participate in our own wellness returns. If you are unable to take one of these gut microbiome tests, then just get to know your body and see what foods make you feel good and which ones don't. I have always felt that there is not one food path to wellness; there are many paths and they are individual.

And check this out: You can also do a gut microbiome test on your pet. If your animal companion has tummy issues, you may want to check this test out. My good friend has a dog with inflammatory bowel disease, and she is healing his gut by shifting his food. My dog Jack McCormick has a sensitive tummy, too (and he's been known to drink out of our toilet bowl—the mecca of the external microbiome!) Similarly, when our cattle get the bovine version of Crohn's disease (called John's disease), we treat it by shifting their gut biome with probiotics and minerals.

that regulate histamine in the body: DAO (diamine oxidase) and histamine N-methyltransferase (HNMT). Missing these enzymes meant she was having a histamine overflow.

Histamines are chemicals in our bodies that produce a natural response to allergens. Our bodies produce white blood cells called *mast cells* to release histamine during an inflammatory-immune response to whatever we are allergic to. This is part of a balanced and healthy immune system. Lots of foods contain histamines and trigger the release of these histamines in the body. When there is a deficiency of the enzymes that break them down—DAO and HNMT—the body gets slammed with an overflow of histamine and has no way to process it. This is histamine intolerance.

Histamine intolerance can get tricky to diagnose because it's basically an allergic reaction without the allergen, sometimes called a "pseudoallergy." The symptoms can vary and may include rashes, breathing problems, runny nose, anxiety, brain fog, digestive distress, eczema, fatigue, hormone imbalances, irritability, low blood pressure, migraines, and nausea after eating. I get migraines and digestive distress when my microbiome is out of balance and I've overindulged in high-histamine foods. But as I have brought my gut back into balance, the migraines are less frequent, the nausea is rare, and my digestive distress is less.

Histamine intolerance can be caused by small intestinal bacterial overgrowth (SIBO), leaky gut, gluten sensitivity, medications (antibiotics, NSAIDS, and pain medications), methylation impairments, and mastocytosis, which leads to many mast cells. To know for sure, consult a functional medicine specialist.

What to Do & What Not to Eat

If you have or suspect that you have histamine intolerance, here are some suggestions:

- See a qualified functional medicine specialist, and get tested for a high histamine/DAO ratio.

- Learn everything you can about histamine intolerance and low-histamine foods.

- Avoid high-histamine foods including alcohol, bone broth, canned foods, cheese (including goat cheese), chocolate, eggplant, legumes, mushrooms, processed foods, smoked meats (bacon, sausage, lunch meat, etc.), shellfish, spinach, and all vinegars. Say goodbye to leftovers; as food sits, it naturally gathers histamines (immediately freeze leftovers). Energy drinks and teas (black, green, and yerba) are also triggers for folks with histamine intolerance or sensitivity. All fermented foods and mushrooms are off the table—*for now*. While they are good for the gut in general, until the histamine intolerance is reversed, they need to be avoided. Avocado, bananas, citrus fruits, kiwi, plums, strawberries, and tomatoes are low histamine but can still trigger the release of histamine, so they are also best avoided.

- There are histamine-free probiotics for people with histamine intolerance, which can help rebuild the gut. You might want to check those out.

- Black cumin and quercetin have antihistamine properties. Ask your functional medicine doctor to find out if they are a fit for you.

- Try the elimination diet to see how you feel. Here's a link to the guidelines: *https://www.his taminintoleranz.ch/downloads/SIGHI-Leaflet_HistamineEliminationDiet.pdf*. Even though the low-histamine diet seems rigid and limited, know that once you build back the good gut bacteria, the possibility of reintroducing histamine foods and not having a problem with them is the goal.

- Be sure to add back foods you hadn't been eating to restore balance to the gut, including non-citrus fruits, veggies (except tomatoes, eggplants, and spinach), coconut milk, egg yolk, fresh wild-caught fish, fresh organic meats, gluten-free grains (rice and corn), fresh fruits, and rice milk. Plus, the DAO enzyme requires vitamin B6, vitamin C, and copper, which many of these foods contain.

Wheat/Gluten Sensitivity and Intolerance

Even in healthy people, processed wheat is irritating to the intestinal tract, and those with weak digestion struggle even more. And here's a double whammy: Processed wheat contains pesticides. Many believe that all these chemicals and additives are wearing down our immune system as it tries to combat these foreign agents, leading to high numbers of wheat allergies, such as celiac disease and gluten sensitivity.

Gluten is best compared to glue, 'cause that is what it does naturally in breads and grains containing gluten: it keeps it all together. Too much slows down the intestinal tract and irritates it. Removing it from the diet has been known to help folks with inflammatory conditions such as arthritis and asthma, as well as autoimmune diseases and even attention deficit disorder.

When I was suffering digestive distress, I underwent a slew of tests, including a blood test for celiac disease, which came back negative. The doctor said there was no reason to avoid gluten, so I continued to eat it. After suffering for many more months, another doctor told me I could be "gluten sensitive." It made sense because I had all the symptoms after I would eat something with gluten—bloating, gas, abdominal pain, nausea, occasional headaches, brain fog, fatigue, and joint pain. (These symptoms can be the same with celiac disease).

There are currently no methods to test for non-celiac gluten sensitivity. Some functional medi-cine doctors offer blood, saliva, or stool testing, but these tests have not been validated, since no antibodies in the blood are specific enough or sensitive enough to show non-celiac gluten sensitivity. Scientists are now making biomarkers to test for non-celiac gluten sensitivity, which will be fantastic because when you are told you are just gluten sensitive as opposed to full-blown celiac, you become less strict about eating gluten. At least that's what I did. If you think you are gluten sensitive, there's no reason to keep eating it. There are many great gluten-free alternatives for your favorite recipes, as you'll discover in Part Three of this book.

When I was told that I was "only gluten sensitive," I thought a little gluten wouldn't hurt. So, I'd have a gluten-free bun with my bean burger, but I'd sneak a few fries that I knew came out of the gluten-filled fryer. When my kids ordered gluten-laden desserts, I'd sneak a bite or two. The server would look at me like, "Oh my gosh, another fake gluten-free person." But, at that time, nobody really knew the health implications; not even the doctors knew. What I did know for sure was that if I ate an entire gluten bun, I'd be in tons of pain.

"Gluten Free" Doesn't Mean Healthy

When I gave up gluten entirely, I did what most people do: I immediately cut out gluten and shifted to gluten-free products, ignoring what was in them because I was psyched that they didn't contain gluten. However, what *is* in most gluten-free products is sugar, yeast, and some dairy. Gluten sensitivity or celiac disease, which is an autoimmune response creating an allergy to gluten, shows itself by creating irritation of the intestinal lining, causing tummy aches, gas, bloating, pressure, constipation, and diarrhea.

Gluten-free products, if they are full of sugar, dairy, and yeast, are still doing damage. Not knowing any of this, I moved right on to the gluten-free muffin and gluten-free bread "plan," not realizing that the majority of gluten-free foods I was eating were packed with fiber-less starches, xanthan gum (which can bother some people), refined sugars, and baking soda packed with aluminum. (Breads made with these ingredients are referred to as "soda pop" bread.) Now that I am better educated, I still eat gluten-free foods; I just learned to read the labels. If they are packed with sugar and unhealthy gluten-free grains, I pass or limit my intake.

If you're healing your digestive tract, be mindful to purchase gluten-free products that are organic to avoid pesticides and genetically modified organisms (GMOs).

Celiac Disease

Celiac disease is a serious autoimmune disorder triggered by consuming gluten protein, which is found in wheat, barley, and rye. When folks with celiac eat gluten, the protein interferes with the absorption of nutrients from food and damages the villi in the small intestines. Damaged villi can't absorb nutrients into the bloodstream, leading to malnourishment and a host of other problems, including some cancers, thyroid disease, infertility, and the onset of other autoimmune diseases. Because the microbiome is wrecked as a result of celiac, it has to be rebuilt—but gently.

One out of 133 Americans has celiac disease; that's equivalent to 1 percent of the U.S. population. Unfortunately, 8 percent of the 3 million Americans living with celiac remain undiagnosed or misdiagnosed.[34] Celiac has been believed to be a genetic disorder passed down from parent to child. However, now that we are understanding autoimmune disease better, we are learning that it doesn't have to be passed down. The body has a tipping point based on stress, emotional trauma, environmental triggers, infection, diet, and even surgery.

Celiac left unattended leads to ulcerations, which can lead to Crohn's disease or colitis, or severe inflammation and ulcerations of the digestive tract. People with Crohn's disease and colitis don't themselves have celiac, but they can have a difficult time digesting glutens and, particularly, wheat. Most folks just remove the gluten and don't know to take steps to heal the damage that the gluten sensitivity has done.

Knowledge Is Power

Two months ago, as of this writing, I tested positive for celiac disease and Hashimoto's disease. Celiac leads to thyroid disease. I now know that dipping my hand in those fries hurt me more than I was prepared for. Now, of course, I am better educated. I pretty much only eat out in Pinewood Kitchen because my team is so dang caring. The good news is, knowledge is power, and food can be medicine. Despite my diagnosis, I still wake up every day full of energy (sometimes I'm even up with the roosters). I'm physically able to work on the farm, be goofy with my girls, and dance with my cowboy husband to our live jam sessions on Saturday nights. I do not think I'd be this healthy if it were not for the real food I've been putting into my body.

I do my best to incorporate all this information and research into my daily menu at Pinewood Kitchen. The recipes that I put together are vast and different, and my goal is to find something for everyone, and to take classic recipes and make them even more delicious and digestible. Feel free to tweak the recipes in this book so that you and your family can eat them based on *your* individual preferences and *your* individual microbiomes.

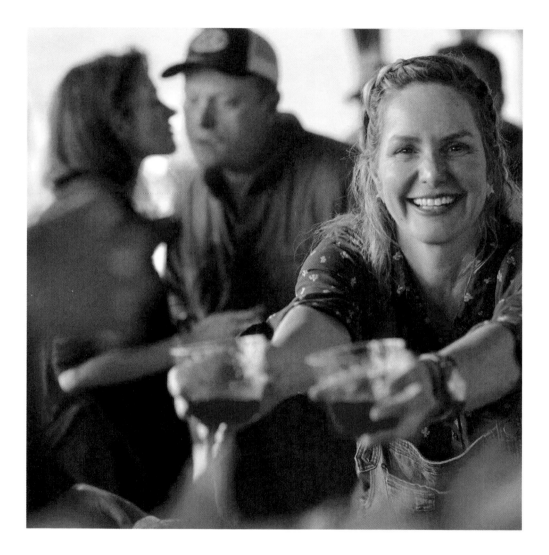

Cheers to Your Health!

Part Three

Let's Eat—The Recipes

My goal with these recipes is to be as inclusive as possible—even if you take away just a handful of gut-healthy recipes for your particular microbiome, then I have done my job. Your goal is to listen to your body and have fun experimenting with foods that may be new to you or reimagining your old favorites. But before you begin, let me give you a little know-how when it comes to cooking with gluten-free flour, butter, grains, beans, and sea vegetables. Once you've got the info, you can make these recipes with confidence.

Whatcha Need to Know

All the recipes in this book are gluten free. When making them, be sure to use 1-to-1 gluten-free flour blends. Bob's Red Mill Gluten Free 1-to-1 Baking Flour has a base of sweet white rice flour, brown rice flour, and potato starch. The mild rice flavor is a neutral and complementary base for most sweet recipes. It also has the sorghum and tapioca flour added along with the addition of xanthan gum. With the xanthan gum already blended into this mixture, it can be a simple cup-for-cup replacement in most baking recipes.

Aside from the occasional call for butter or goat cheese, these recipes are dairy free. I also give you the choice of what type of butter you want to use and what works for you and your body. I am allergic to dairy, so I use vegan butter. Ghee, which is clarified butter, is easier to digest because the fats that can cause a digestive reaction are removed. Ghee can be used in place of olive oil at times.

If you are fine with butter, then I suggest using grass-fed butter. If you are dairy-free and a recipe calls for goat cheese, you'll find that ricotta made from almonds is an excellent substitute. If you don't eat eggs, you'll even find egg replacement recipes. Some of these recipes are labeled "vegan," which simply means the recipe is dairy free, egg free, meat free, and honey free.

About the Substitutions

I've included substitutions in the ingredients list from time to time not only to give you a choice but also to get you thinking about how you can personalize these recipes. This doesn't mean these are the only substitutions you can make, and it certainly doesn't mean that you can't substitute ingredients in recipes that don't specify substitutions. For instance, if dairy is okay for you, go ahead and use dairy milk if you want to. If you can't eat cashews, try a different nut or seeds. If you're watching your salt intake, use less salt or omit it (unless you're baking something for which the amount of salt specified is necessary for the finished product). You are totally free to use your imagination and cooking experience to make these recipes uniquely suited to your body.

Equivalents	
I have this little chart taped to the inside of my cupboard so I always know how to break down my measuring.	
3 teaspoons (tsp.) = 1 tablespoon (tbsp.)	4 tbsp. = ¼ cup
5⅓ tbsp. = ⅓ cup	16 tbsp. = 1 cup
1 cup = 8 fluid ounces (fl. oz.) = ½ pint (pt.)	2 cups = 1 pt.
4 cups = ¼ gallon (gal.) = 1 quart (qt.)	4 cups = 1 liter (L)—roughly
5 milliliters (mL) = 1 tsp.	125 mL = ½ cup
250 mL = 1 cup	946 mL = 4 cups
1.89 liters (L) = 8 cups	28 (g.) = 1 (oz.)
100 grams (g.) = 3½ ounces (oz.)	454 g. = 1 (lb.)
16 oz. = 1 pound (lb.)	

The Rules of Beans

Beans are no joke when it comes to being good fo' ya! I had been told by every doctor I'd met that it wouldn't be possible for someone with my intestinal issues to ever eat beans. Well, that turned out to be a myth, 'cause I get down with these little protein packers. Don't forget that beans are cheap, and they go a long way! Here are some rules for preparing beans:

- Soak dried beans overnight in water with kombu sea vegetable. (If you can't find kombu in your market or health food store, kombu and all sea veggies can be ordered online and delivered to your door.) Be sure to drain and rinse the beans after soaking, and then add new water before cooking.

- Remove and rinse the kombu after soaking—I usually chop mine up into pieces before adding it back to the cooking pot.

- Be mindful that beans come from the ground, where they are among rocks and dirt. Go through your beans before you cook them, searching for broken beans and tiny stones that could easily have been missed.

- Most beans double in volume from dry to cooked. One cup of dried beans serves about four people. Soybeans and garbanzo beans usually triple.

- Place whole garlic cloves and quarter pieces of onion into the cooking pot. (Don't chop up the onion or garlic or they will get scooped out when you skim the foam.)

- Bring your beans to a boil, which helps the beans really pop, and then cover, and reduce heat to a simmer for 30 minutes.

- Remove the sponge-like foam that floats to the top of the pot while cooking. This foam is home to the gas-causing carbohydrates. If you don't remove it, your tummy will fo'sho be in a state of methane suffering!

- Add salt *during the last 10 minutes of cooking*. If you add salt any sooner, it will slow the cooking time.

Cooking Beans, Lentils & Peas (AKA Legumes)

The key to cooking beans is to be sure you've cooked them thoroughly. Where folks go wrong is turning off the stove too soon. If they aren't done in the recommended time, add more water and turn up the heat, bringing them to a boil for another 15 minutes. Cook legumes in lots of water, then drain afterward (except lentils and split peas).

Legume	Soaking Time	Water Legumes*	Cooking Time	Nutritional Values and Additional Notes
Aduki (adzuki) beans	2–4 hours	3:1	1–1½ hours	Easy to digest; tones kidneys according to traditional Chinese medicine
Black beans	6–12 hours	4:1	1½ hours	Contains the most antioxidants of any legume
Black-eyed peas	4–12 hours	3:1	1 hour	Protein, minerals, B vitamins, and isoflavones
Cannellini (white kidney) beans	6–12 hours	3:1	1–1½ hours	Molybdenum, folate, and tryptophan
Chickpeas (garbanzo beans)	6–12 hours	4:1	2 hours	Contains more iron than any other legume; protein and molybdenum
Kidney beans	6–12 hours	3:1	1½–2 hours	Molybdenum, folate, tryptophan, and protein
Lima beans	6–12 hours	2:1	1½ hours	Molybdenum and tryptophan
Lentils	20 minutes–4 hours	3:1	45–60 minutes	Molybdenum, folate, and tryptophan; easy to digest (less gassy); second highest amount of protein of any legume
Navy beans	4–12 hours	3:1	1–1½ hours	Tryptophan, folate, and manganese; controls blood sugar

Pinto beans	6–12 hours	3:1	1½ hours	Molybdenum, folate, and tryptophan
Soybeans	6–12 hours	4:1	3–5 hours	Highest amount of protein of any legume (can be difficult to digest though); molybdenum, tryptophan, and manganese

*ratio of water to legumes

The Rules of Grains

We were a rigatoni pasta family, and my momma didn't like rice 'cause her momma didn't make it. In fact, I never once ate whole grains growing up. As an adult, I never ate any grains other than an occasional side of brown rice. I didn't know what I was missing.

There is a lot of talk that eating grains is contributing to the demise of the intestinal lining, but if you soak them and cook them properly and eat them in whole form, they can be part of a balanced diet. I healed the ulceration in my intestines and ate grains and legumes twice a week. (However, if you are suffering from digestive distress or a flare-up, only eat brown rice or millet until your digestive tract has calmed down.)

It's also become fashionable to avoid all carbohydrates and grains, as a part of several trendy fad diets. Sadly, this theory is wrong. Eating whole grains in moderation and rotating them along with plenty of vegetables is the key to balancing the body.

Whole grains are best used in their original form with all their parts intact: the bran, the germ, and the endosperm. When manufacturers remove the bran and germ to make refined flour, they remove most of the vitamins and minerals—a major no-no if you want to get good nutrition out of them. If you follow these rules, grain intimidation is no longer an issue:

- I soak all my grains overnight (except millet and quinoa), and if you are suffering from digestive troubles, it's a good idea to do that. Be sure to add a two-inch piece of kombu sea vegetable when soaking. The kombu helps cut the carbohydrates that cause gas, and it adds minerals to your grains—boost 'em, baby!

- You do not have to soak millet or quinoa overnight. Instead, it is recommended you soak them for 20 minutes and then rinse them. Be sure to toss your kombu into the pot with your grains. I also hydrate an extra two-inch piece of kombu and dice it up. Then I add it to my grains just before serving; this way I'm sure to get all the minerals in my bowl.

- After soaking, rinse your grains, and add fresh water to your cooking pot. The soaking water is full of grain garbage: excess gas-causing carbohydrates and dirt!

- The key to cooking grains that taste yummy is making sure you've cooked them long enough (see the chart below). If you are suffering from any type of digestive distress or are healing your body and need to aid absorption, add extra water to make the grains more like a porridge. After you've made these grains a few times, you'll have a rhythm for it, and the timing will come naturally.

Cooking Grains

Grain	Water: Grain*	Cooking Time	Approximate Yield**	Nutritional Values and Additional Notes
Amaranth	2:1	20–30 minutes	2 cups	Very high in fiber, protein, and calcium; easy to digest
Buckwheat	2:1	10–15 minutes	2 cups	Lowers risk of high cholesterol and high blood pressure
Cornmeal	3:1	30 minutes	3 cups	B vitamins, which support lung health, memory, and energy when under stress
Millet	2:1	20–30 minutes	3½–4 cups	Most alkalinizing grain
Oats (whole)†	2¼:1	½–1 hour	2–2½ cups	Nourishes nervous system
Oats (rolled)†	2:1	5–10 minutes	4 cups	Nourishes nervous system

Quinoa	2:1	15–30 minutes	3–3½ cups	Highest protein of any grain; more calcium than cow's milk; contains vitamins B, E, and iron
Rice, brown	2:1	25–35 minutes	3 cups	Manganese, selenium, magnesium, and B vitamins
Rice, wild	2–4:1	45 minutes	4 cups	Manganese, selenium, magnesium, and B vitamins

*ratio of water to grain in cups
**based on 1 cup dry grain

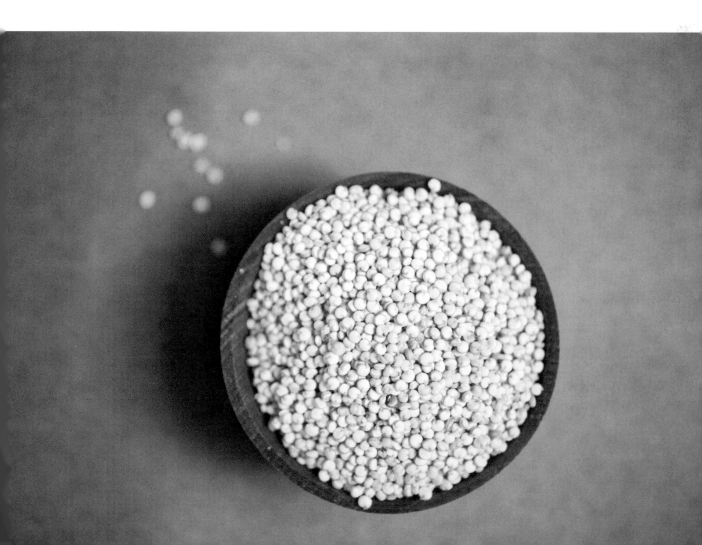

The Wonderful World of Grains

In the beginning of my food journey, I only knew about brown rice, and truth be told, I didn't like it. Most people half cook it, leaving it chewy and tough. Once I was on my new food path, I was in awe of the bulk foods section at Whole Foods. Literally. A world opened up to me, one that would keep my dinner table from ever becoming drab with the same old white rice. Here are some to get comfy with:

Amaranth is not a true cereal grass but a weedy plant of the pigweed family. The seed is high in protein and about the size of a poppy seed. The leaves of amaranth can also be eaten as well. The blooms of the plant are unique and beautiful, with purple, orange, red, or gold colors. In Mexico, amaranth is common in snack bars and cookies. *(Tip: Add amaranth when cooking other grains—about a teaspoon—for added nutrients and flavor.)*

Buckwheat is a cereal unrelated to wheat. After it has been cooked and prepared pilaf-style, it is called kasha. I love buckwheat for baking. It's super yummy, and as a whole grain, it has a distinct fragrant flavor. It's a great gut game-changer to serve at dinner parties. I also love buckwheat porridge and pancakes.

Oats are mechanically pressed or rolled for oatmeal. They can be ground as well. Make sure they are processed in a gluten-free facility and that they are truly 100% gluten free.

Wild rice is not actually a member of the rice family, although it is a grain-producing grass. Native to North America, wild rice can still be found growing wild in the ponds and lakes of Wisconsin, as well as in neighboring states. Native Americans were the first to introduce it to the colonists. Like rice, wild rice grows in water, although it tends to require much deeper water resources. The two grains also have taste similarities: both taste much nuttier with the outer husk left on.

Cookin' with Sea Veggies

The nutritional value of sea vegetables is off the charts—they are the last of the veggies to contain high levels of trace minerals and the broadest range of minerals of *any food*. Folks in Asia and other coastal regions including Ireland, Scotland, Norway, Iceland, and New Zealand have been eating these veggies for 10,000 years. The list of goodies they pack is extensive—from iodine (keeps the thyroid in check), magnesium, calcium (we don't have to drink milk to get it), and zinc to B vitamins, vitamin K, and a good amount of lignans (plant compounds with cancer-protective properties). Sea vegetables—especially hijiki, kombu, and wakame—also contain sodium alginate, which neutralizes and helps eliminate radioactive particles and heavy metals from the body.

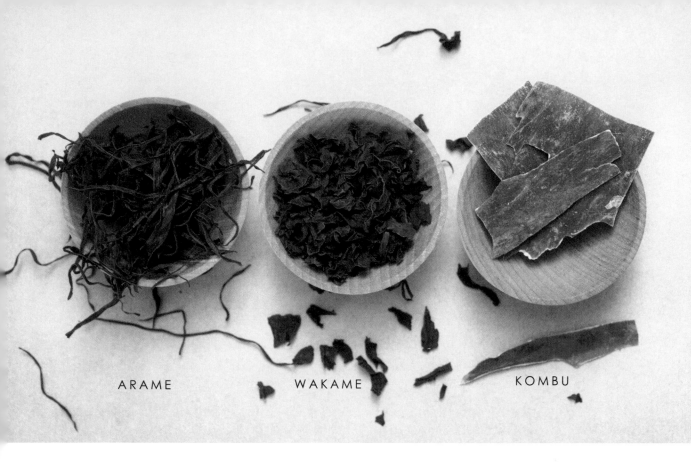

ARAME   WAKAME   KOMBU

The real dealio is that folks who frequently eat seaweed have incredibly lower rates of colon cancer. If you've got a digestive situation, cancer, or a hormonal disruption, get your sea veggies! Since sea vegetables are concentrated foods, you only need to eat a small amount of them—1 to 2 tablespoons per serving—to derive their enormous benefits. The easiest intro to seaweed is to add it to any miso or soup base. As you've read, I add kombu seaweed to my grains and beans while soaking and cooking them to add minerals to my food. You can presoak seaweed, or cut it up and use it in soups or in stir-fries. While there are more than seventy-five species of sea vegetables eaten around the world, the following are some common varieties, their unique qualities, and cooking suggestions:

- **Agar-agar.** These crystal slices of algae are used as a thickener and base in custards, Jell-O, and mousses. Agar-agar (or just agar) is a natural gelatin, best used in flake form. The flakes have no taste or aroma. You simply need to heat them in your liquid of choice and they will dissolve. Usually 1 tablespoon of agar flakes per 1 cup of liquid is needed to create a gel state, or "kanten," as it is called. Agar-agar provides necessary bulk for regulating the intestines.

- **Arame.** Arame is a tasty black vegetable that comes in thin slivers or strands. It has a sweet flavor that is wonderful when cooked with other vegetables, such as carrots or onions. Prepare arame by soaking it to remove any sand or dirt. Once it's rehydrated, lift it out of the remaining water, and add a small amount of the arame to a stir-fry recipe, soup, or stew. Arame can also be cooked alone, or with carrots, onions, or lemon juice, for 30 minutes. Arame is rich in vitamins A and B, carbohydrates, calcium, and trace elements.

- **Dulse.** Dulse is high in iron, rich in protein and vitamins A, C, E, and B, and has iodine and trace elements. It has a tangy, salty flavor that complements vegetables, grains, stews, and fruit dishes. Dry roasted, it becomes a crunchy, savory condiment. Prepare dulse by wiping it with a damp towel to remove any excess salt and sand. Spread it on a cooking sheet and place it in a 250°F oven for 10 minutes.

- **Hijiki.** Hijiki has a robust flavor and bold appearance. It is a stringlike vegetable that is eaten as a side dish. Leftover hijiki is excellent in salads. Prepare hijiki by soaking a small amount in water for about 10 minutes, or until it is rehydrated and soft. Lift it out of the water rather than pouring the water off to allow any residues to settle to the bottom of the bowl. Then boil it alone or with carrots, onions, daikon radish, or beans for 1 to 1½ hours. Hijiki is high in nutrients, especially protein, the B vitamins, vitamin A, calcium, phosphorous, iron, and many trace elements. It is traditionally used to strengthen the bones and to revitalize the skin and hair. It also helps build strong intestines.

- **Irish moss.** Irish moss is a sea vegetable used to thicken soups and stews. It is high in vitamins A and B, iron, sodium, calcium, and other elements.

- **Kombu.** Kombu is a stalklike sea vegetable used to add sweetness and hardiness to dishes. Use it in soups or cook it as a vegetable with carrots, onions, rutabagas, turnips, or daikon radish. When added to vegetables, beans, or grains, it greatly enhances their flavor, as well as softens them and increases their digestibility. In addition, its nutrients leach out during cooking and infuse the other foods. Prepare kombu by rinsing it in water. It can be used in whole form or chopped into small pieces. When soaked or added to soup, it will expand. When used in dishes that are cooked longer, it usually dissolves.

- **Nori.** Nori and sushi nori is the easiest sea vegetable to use and the one that newcomers to sea vegetables enjoy instantly. Nori, which comes in sheets, is commonly eaten in Japanese restaurants and used to wrap sushi. It can be roasted over an open flame in less than a minute and crumpled up to make a condiment. It is loaded with nutrients, including vitamins A, B, C, and D, calcium, phosphorous, iron, and trace elements.

- **Wakame.** Wakame is good in miso and other soups and stews. It enriches the flavor of other vegetables, such as carrots or onions. It can also be used as a sweetener. It is leafy and slippery in texture and expands when it is soaked, so one "square" is enough. It is best when soaked, chopped, and added to soups. When boiled, it is fully cooked in twenty minutes. Loaded with nutrients, wakame is high in calcium, thiamine, niacin, and vitamin B. It is traditionally used in Chinese medicine to purify the blood and strengthen the skin, hair, and intestines.

Build Your Own Buddha Bowl

If you have leftover beans, grains, and/or vegetables, whip up a Buddha Bowl, as we call 'em in Pinewood. You can jazz up the flavors by drizzling the top with homemade ranch (see page 73) or sweet chili sauce (see page 223) or use a gluten-free store-bought sauce. When my digestive system was healing, Buddha Bowls were my go-to meal, and they are great to have on hand in the fridge for the kids to eat instead of fast food.

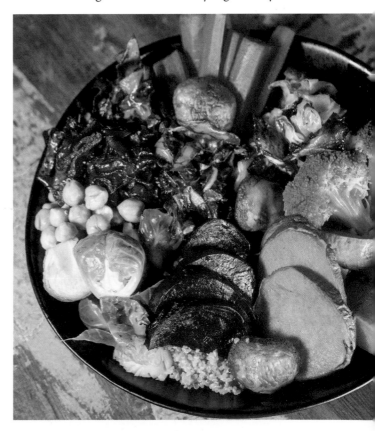

Now that you've got all that info under your belt, it's time to get cookin'! We'll start with some of my favorite salads and soups, and then get creative with the main event along with delish side dishes and veggies. Following that, you'll learn how to make yummy sauces and dips, and then we'll top it all off with gluten-free breads and sweets. Hold on to your chef hat, 'cause here we go!

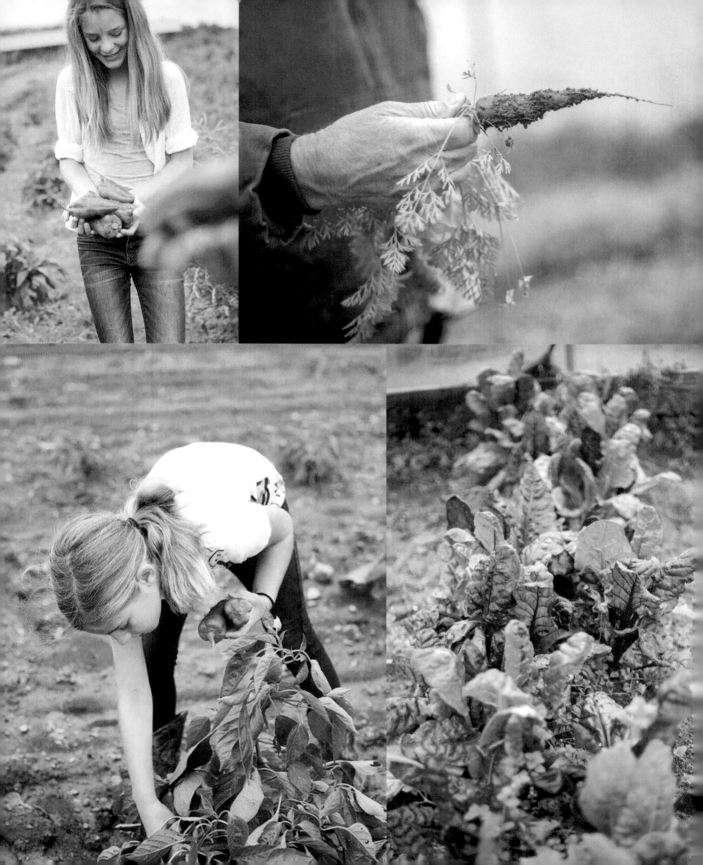

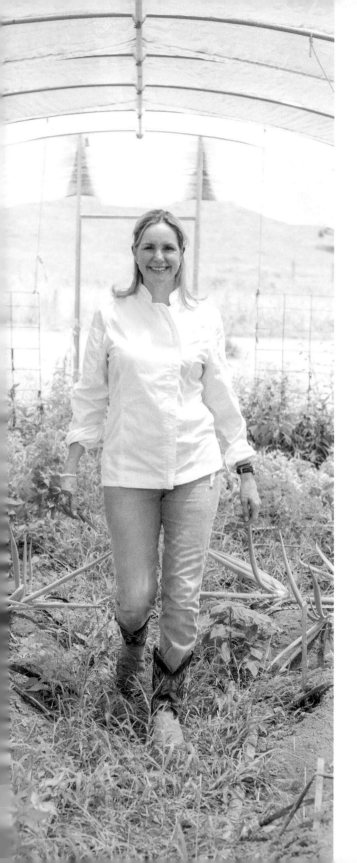

Supa Salads

We grow a variety of salad greens in Pinewood and I love a crispy, cool bite of goodness. I find salads are a great way to support a diverse gut culture by tossing everything together, and my salad ingredients shift easily with whatever we have available off the farm or from other local farmers.

I am mindful of my digestion, and when it's weak, I lean toward eating cooked veggies and my beloved Buddha Bowl is my go-to dish as we rotate what we have off the farm.

Substitutions:

*If meat free, replace with Coconut Bacon *(page 157)* or *Tempeh Bacon *(page 158)*.

**If egg free, omit the eggs.

***If meat free, replace with grilled portobello mushrooms.

The Ranch Hand Salad

Makes 4 servings

FOR THE RANCH DRESSING:

1 tablespoon fresh lemon juice *or* apple cider vinegar

¼ cup unsweetened oat milk, organic soy milk, *or* other nondairy milk

1 cup Vegan Mayo *(page 213)*

1 teaspoon garlic powder

1 teaspoon onion powder

¼ teaspoon sea salt

Freshly ground black pepper *(to taste)*

2 teaspoons chopped fresh parsley *(optional)*

½ teaspoon chopped fresh dill *or* ¼ teaspoon dried dill

FOR THE SALAD:

1 large bunch Lacinato kale *(Tuscan kale)*, stems removed and chopped into bite-size pieces

4 ounces watercress, torn into bite-size pieces

3 *(6-ounce)* boneless, skinless chicken breasts, cooked and chopped*

10 ounces grape tomatoes, halved

2 avocados, halved, pitted, and cut into ½-inch pieces

3 large farm eggs, hard-cooked and cut into ½-inch pieces**

2 ounces goat cheese *or* almond milk ricotta, crumbled

3 tablespoons minced fresh chives

8 slices cooked bacon, cut into ¼-inch pieces***

Sea salt *(to taste)*

Freshly ground black pepper *(to taste)*

TO MAKE THE DRESSING:

1) In a small bowl, whisk together the lemon juice with the milk; let the mixture sit for a couple of minutes to create your dairy-free "buttermilk."

2) Place the remaining ingredients in a blender or food processor. Add the "buttermilk" and blend until silky smooth and creamy.

TO MAKE THE SALAD:

1) In a large bowl, combine the kale and watercress with 5 tablespoons of the dressing and toss to coat; arrange over a flat serving platter.

2) Add the chopped chicken to the bowl and toss with a ¼ cup of the dressing; arrange the chicken in a row along one edge of the greens.

3) Add the tomatoes to the bowl and toss with 1 tablespoon of the dressing; arrange the tomatoes on the opposite edge of greens.

4) In separate rows near the center of the greens, arrange the avocados and eggs. Drizzle with the remaining dressing. Sprinkle the cheese, chives, and bacon evenly over the salad. Season with salt and pepper and serve.

BLUEBERRIES ARE TRULY ONE OF THE BEST THINGS WE CAN ALL EAT
a couple of times a week. Luckily, during the season, our blueberry bushes bring our tiny kitchen bushels of abundance. We make this salad at least once a week when blueberries are in season. Folks are always super impressed, and I tell them this is the easiest salad you will ever make. I love adding leftover quinoa to salads because it gives it something extra in terms of taste, texture, and nutrition. You can also skip the goat cheese and chicken and toss in cooked chickpeas and apple slices—YUM!

Blueberry Almond Salad

Makes 4 servings

FOR THE DRESSING:

½ cup fresh blueberries

¼ cup rice vinegar

1 teaspoon lemon zest

4 tablespoons lemon juice

3 tablespoons local honey*

¾ cup extra-virgin olive oil

Sea salt *(to taste)*

Freshly ground black pepper *(to taste)*

Substitutions:

*If watching sugar, use an equivalent amount of stevia *(page 51)*.

FOR THE SALAD:

6 cups mixed greens

1½ cups fresh blueberries

¼ cup finely sliced red onions

½ cup toasted almonds

2 grilled chicken breasts, chopped *(optional)***

½ cup cooked quinoa *(optional)*

¼ cup goat cheese *or* almond cheese, crumbled

Substitutions:

**If meat free, replace with sliced avocado.

1) Place the dressing ingredients in a blender or food processor and puree until smooth. Season with salt and pepper to taste.

2) In a medium bowl, toss together the greens, blueberries, onions, almonds, chicken (if using), and quinoa (if using). Top with the cheese and drizzle with the dressing. Serve immediately.

Black Rice Salad with Snap Peas and Ginger–Sesame Vinaigrette

Makes 4 servings

ANTIOXIDANT-RICH BLACK RICE—ONCE CONSIDERED FOOD FOR NOBLES—IS NOW available to all. The hull contains large amounts of anthocyanin, which is also found in blueberries and red cabbage. The hull is gut-lovin' food for our gut bacteria. I make black rice in advance and then whip this up when I have leftover veggies.

4 quarts water

1½ cups black rice

1 teaspoon plus ¼ teaspoon sea salt

1 teaspoon plus 3 tablespoons rice vinegar

2 teaspoons minced shallot

1½ tablespoons local honey

2 teaspoons Sweet Chili Sauce *(page 223)*

1 teaspoon grated fresh ginger

⅛ teaspoon black pepper

¼ cup extra-virgin olive oil

1 tablespoon toasted sesame oil

6 ounces sugar snap peas, strings removed, and halved

5 radishes, trimmed, halved, and sliced thin

1 red bell pepper, stemmed, seeded, and chopped fine

¼ cup minced fresh cilantro

1) In a large pot over medium-high heat, bring the water to a boil. Add the rice and 1 teaspoon of the sea salt and cover. Cook until the rice is tender, about 20 to 25 minutes.

2) Drain the rice, spread onto a rimmed baking sheet, drizzle with 1 teaspoon of the vinegar, and let it cool for 15 minutes.

3) In a large bowl, whisk together the shallots, honey, Sweet Chili Sauce, ginger, the remaining sea salt, black pepper, and the remaining 3 tablespoons vinegar. Whisking slowly, drizzle in the olive oil and sesame oil until combined.

4) Add the cooled rice, snap peas, radishes, bell pepper, and cilantro, and toss to combine. Season with additional sea salt and pepper to taste, if desired, and serve.

Tabbouleh Cauliflower Salad

Makes 4 servings

I AM A TABBOULEH

kinda gal. Once you fall in love with tabbouleh, you will crave it. Finding ways to load my body with parsley is a goal, and this recipe is my go-to. You can make this with leftover quinoa or buy bagged riced cauliflower from your local market.

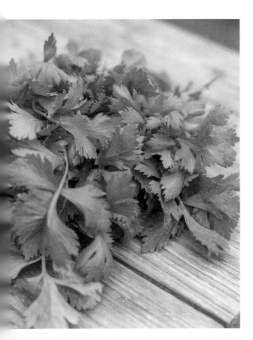

½ medium head cauliflower, coarsely chopped

2 cups packed flat-leaf parsley leaves

1 cup mint leaves

2 scallions, thinly sliced

1 clove garlic, chopped

1 teaspoon lemon zest

3 tablespoons fresh lemon juice

1 teaspoon sea salt

5 tablespoons extra-virgin olive oil

¼ teaspoon crushed red pepper flakes *(optional)*

½ medium cucumber, cut into ¼-inch pieces

6 ounces cherry tomatoes, quartered

1) Place the chopped cauliflower in a food processor and pulse for about 30 seconds. Don't pulse too much, or you will have mushy cauliflower. The pieces should look like chunky rice. Wipe out the food processor to remove the cauliflower remnants.

2) You don't have to cook the cauliflower, but if your digestion is wonky like mine, hit it in a hot skillet for 4 minutes, just until toasted. Be careful not to overcook it.

3) In the food processor, combine the parsley, mint, scallions, garlic, lemon zest, lemon juice, salt, and olive oil. Pulse until the herbs are coarsely chopped.

4) In a large bowl, toss together the cauliflower, red pepper flakes (if using), cucumber, tomatoes, and herb mixture, and serve.

I AM A SUCKA FO' SUCCOTASH. WE HAVE A SAYING IN THE RESTAURANT AND ON THE farm: If it grows together, it goes together—and that's exactly what this salad is: the perfect match.

Farmhouse Succotash Salad with Avocado Dressing

Makes 4 servings

2 ears fresh corn, husks and silks removed

1 cup fresh *or* frozen lima beans

¾ cup oat milk *or* other nondairy milk

3 teaspoons apple cider vinegar, divided

½ avocado, pitted and peeled

1 tablespoon chopped fresh Italian parsley

1 small clove garlic, minced

¼ teaspoon sea salt

¼ teaspoon onion powder

¼ teaspoon dry mustard

¼ teaspoon black pepper

1 large head of butter lettuce, torn

2 cups sliced grilled chicken breast*

½ cup finely chopped red onion

½ cup crumbled goat cheese *or* almond milk ricotta

6 slices crispy bacon, crumbled**

Substitutions:

*If meat free, replace with grilled portobello mushrooms.

**If meat free, replace with a handful of toasted pecans.

1) Cut the kernels from the cobs and discard the cobs.

2) In a small pan, cook lima beans in lightly salted boiling water for about 15 minutes or until tender. Remove with a slotted spoon. Set aside.

3) Add the corn kernels to the boiling water and cook for about 5 minutes. Set aside.

4) In a medium bowl, whisk together the milk and the apple cider vinegar. Allow it to sit for a few minutes to create dairy-free "buttermilk."

5) In a blender or food processor, combine the avocado, parsley, garlic, sea salt, onion powder, dry mustard, and black pepper. Then add the "buttermilk." Blend until creamy. If it's too thick, add a little more milk.

6) Arrange the lettuce on a large platter. Arrange the lima beans, corn, chicken, onion, cheese, and bacon in rows over the lettuce and drizzle with the dressing. Alternatively, mix it all up, and serve.

BUTTERNUT SQUASH AND LENTILS ARE A PERFECT COMBO FOR A COOL FALL day. This recipe is comfort food all the way — it's full of flavor and has a satisfying crunch. Lentils, pumpkin seeds, and butternut squash are great for the gut. All the spices in this dish boost our immunity, too.

Spiced Lentil Salad with Butternut Squash

Makes about 4 servings

1¼ teaspoons sea salt, divided

4 cups warm soaking water

1 cup dried black lentils, picked over and rinsed

1 pound butternut squash, peeled, seeded, and cut into ½-inch pieces*

5 tablespoons extra-virgin olive oil, divided

2 tablespoons balsamic vinegar, divided

¼ teaspoon black pepper

1 garlic clove, minced

½ teaspoon ground coriander

¼ teaspoon ground cumin

¼ teaspoon ground ginger

⅛ teaspoon ground cinnamon

4 cups fresh water

1 teaspoon Dijon mustard

½ cup fresh parsley leaves

¼ cup finely chopped red onion

1 tablespoon raw pumpkin seeds, toasted, *or* pepitas

Substitutions:

*If short on time, buy butternut squash that's already peeled and chopped in your produce department.

1) In a medium bowl, dissolve 1 teaspoon of the sea salt in the soaking water. Add the lentils and soak at room temperature for a minimum of 1 hour. Drain well.

2) Adjust the oven racks to the middle and lowest positions and heat the oven to 450°F.

3) Toss the squash with 1 tablespoon of the oil, 1½ teaspoons of the vinegar, the remaining sea salt, and the black pepper. Arrange the squash in a single layer on a rimmed baking sheet and roast on the lower rack until well browned and tender, about 20 to 25 minutes, stirring halfway through roasting. Let the squash cool slightly. Decrease the oven temperature to 325°F.

4) In a saucepan over medium heat, combine the lentils, 1 tablespoon of the oil, the garlic, coriander, cumin, ginger, and cinnamon; cook until fragrant, about 1 minute. Stir in the 4 cups of water. Cover and simmer for about 40 minutes until the lentils are soft. Drain well.

5) In a large bowl, whisk together the mustard, the remaining oil, and the remaining vinegar. Add the parsley and onion. Toss in the lentils and squash. Season with additional sea salt and pepper, to taste.

6) Transfer to a serving platter and sprinkle with the pumpkin seeds or pepitas. Serve warm or at room temperature.

Crispy Spiced Chickpea Salad with Honey Mustard Vinaigrette

Makes 4 servings

FOR THE SALAD:

1 teaspoon smoked paprika

1 teaspoon coconut sugar *or* stevia

½ teaspoon ground cumin

½ teaspoon sea salt

¼ teaspoon cayenne pepper

¾ cup plus 1 tablespoon olive oil

2 cups soaked, rinsed, and cooked chickpeas*

1 red onion, halved and sliced through the root end

6 cups mixed greens with arugula

FOR THE DRESSING:

1½ tablespoons apple cider vinegar

1 tablespoon whole-grain mustard

2 teaspoons local honey

1½ teaspoons grated lemon zest

¾ teaspoon Basic Mayo *(page 212) or* Vegan Mayo *(page 213)*

¼ teaspoon sea salt

¼ cup extra-virgin olive oil

Substitutions:

*If short on time, replace with 1 (15-ounce) can chickpeas, rinsed and thoroughly dried.

1) In a large bowl, combine the paprika, coconut sugar, cumin, sea salt, and cayenne pepper in a large bowl; set aside.

2) In a large Dutch oven over high heat, heat ¾ cup of the oil until just smoking. Add the chickpeas and onions and partially cover with the lid to prevent splattering; cook, stirring occasionally, until deep golden brown and crispy, about 10 to 12 minutes. Using a slotted spoon, transfer the chickpeas and onions to a paper towel-lined plate and let them drain briefly.

3) In the large bowl with the reserved spice mixture, add the chickpeas and onions, and toss. Let the mixture cool.

4) Add the mixed greens to the chickpea mixture and toss to combine.

5) In a bowl, whisk together the vinegar, mustard, honey, lemon zest, mayo, and sea salt. Whisking constantly, drizzle in the oil.

6) Drizzle the dressing over the salad and toss to combine. Serve immediately.

Tofu and Vegetable Salad

Makes 4 servings

THIS IS AN EXCELLENT INTRODUCTION TO TOFU. THE FRESHNESS OF THE RED BELL pepper, snow peas, and cabbage mixed with tofu creates a party on the plate as tofu absorbs the flavors it's served with. If you don't eat tofu, add grilled chicken or grilled shrimp and it's equally yummy.

1¾ pounds soft tofu, cut into ¾-inch cubes

Sea salt *(to taste)*

Freshly ground black pepper *(to taste)*

3 tablespoons lime juice (about 2 limes)

3 tablespoons local honey

2 tablespoons rice vinegar

2 tablespoons fish sauce, plus extra for serving

1 tablespoon grated fresh ginger

1½ teaspoons sriracha sauce

6 tablespoons extra-virgin olive oil, divided

3 tablespoons toasted sesame oil

4 cups shredded Napa cabbage

6 ounces snow peas, strings removed, cut in half lengthwise

2 carrots, peeled and shredded

1 red bell pepper, stemmed, seeded, and cut into ½-inch pieces

1 cup bean sprouts

2 scallions, thinly sliced

3 tablespoons minced fresh cilantro

1 tablespoon toasted sesame seeds

1) Spread the tofu over a paper towel-lined baking sheet. Let it drain for 20 minutes, and then gently press dry with paper towels. Season with the salt and pepper.

2) In a medium bowl, whisk together the lime juice, honey, vinegar, fish sauce, ginger, and sriracha sauce. Slowly whisk in 4 tablespoons of the olive oil and the sesame oil until incorporated. Measure out ¼ cup of this vinaigrette mixture for dressing the salad and set aside.

3) In a 12-inch nonstick skillet over medium-high heat, heat 1 tablespoon of the olive oil until shimmering. Add half of the tofu and brown lightly on all sides, about 5 minutes; transfer to the bowl with the remaining vinaigrette. Repeat with the remaining 1 tablespoon of olive oil and the remaining tofu. Gently toss the tofu to coat with the vinaigrette and then let it cool completely, about 10 minutes.

4) Combine the cabbage, snow peas, carrots, bell pepper, bean sprouts, and scallions in a large bowl. Drizzle with the reserved vinaigrette and toss to combine. Add the tofu mixture and toss gently to combine. Season with extra fish sauce, to taste. Sprinkle with the cilantro and sesame seeds, and serve.

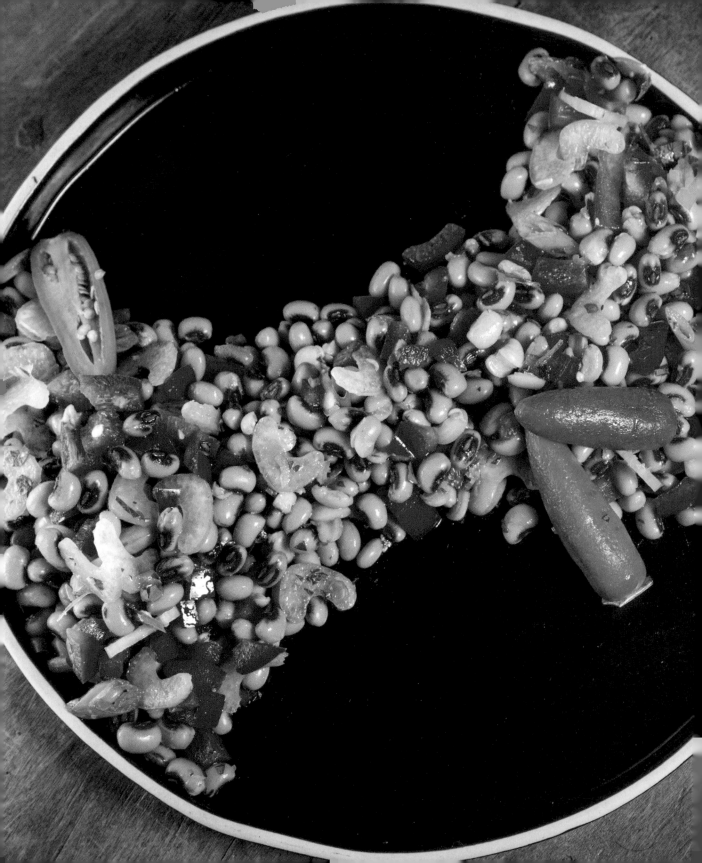

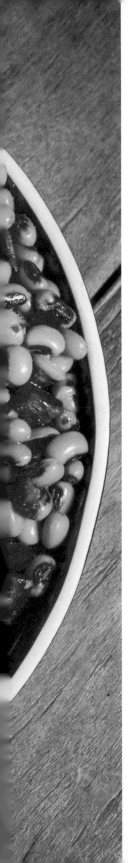

Tennessee Caviar

Makes 4 servings

GARDEN PEAS ARE caviar here in the South. They take a lot of work to pick and shell, and we try to make them the star of the dish so we don't waste the effort. This recipe can be made with any Southern farm pea—purple hull, zipper cream peas, or cow peas. We freeze any peas we don't use right away so we can pull them out on a cold, snowy day, and remember summer isn't that far away.

⅓ cup red wine vinegar

3 tablespoons extra-virgin olive oil

2 garlic cloves, minced

1 teaspoon sea salt plus more *(to taste)*

½ teaspoon pepper plus more *(to taste)*

4 cups soaked, rinsed, and cooked black-eyed peas*

6 scallions, sliced thin

1 red bell pepper, stemmed, seeded, and chopped

1 green bell pepper, stemmed, seeded, and chopped

2 jalapeños, stemmed, seeded, and minced *(optional)*

1 celery rib, chopped fine

¼ cup chopped fresh cilantro

¼ cup chopped fresh parsley

Substitutions:

*If short on time, replace with 2 *(15-ounce)* cans black-eyed peas, rinsed.

1) In a large bowl, whisk together the vinegar, oil, garlic, sea salt, and pepper.

2) Add the peas, scallions, bell peppers, jalapeños (if using), celery, cilantro, and parsley, and toss to combine. Season with sea salt and pepper, to taste.

3) Let sit for at least 1 hour before serving. Tennessee Caviar can be covered and refrigerated for up to five days.

Quinoa Salad with Red Bell Pepper and Cilantro

Makes 4 servings

I MAKE MY QUINOA ahead of time and whip this side salad up right before serving, but you can make it all at once if you prefer. This is a great side dish or as a meal topped with a protein. The hijiki adds selenium and other healthy trace minerals.

1 cup soaked and rinsed white or red quinoa

1½ cups water

¼ teaspoon sea salt

½ red bell pepper, chopped fine

½ jalapeño, minced *(optional)*

2 tablespoons finely chopped red onion

2 tablespoons hydrated hijiki sea vegetable

1 tablespoon minced fresh cilantro

2 tablespoons lime juice

1 tablespoon extra-virgin olive oil

2 teaspoons Dijon mustard

1 garlic clove, minced

½ teaspoon ground cumin

Freshly ground black pepper *(to taste)*

1) Toast the quinoa in a medium saucepan over medium-high heat, stirring frequently until lightly toasted and fragrant, about 5 minutes. Stir in the water and sea salt and bring to a simmer. Decrease the heat to low, cover, and continue to simmer until most of the water has been absorbed and the quinoa is nearly tender, about 16 to 20 minutes.

2) When the quinoa is cool, transfer to a large bowl. Stir in the bell pepper, jalapeño (if using), onion, hijiki, and cilantro.

3) In a separate bowl, whisk together the lime juice, oil, mustard, garlic, and cumin, and then pour over the quinoa mixture and toss to coat. Season with black pepper, to taste, and an additional dash of sea salt, if desired, and serve.

Seaweed Salad

Makes 2 to 4 servings

WAKAME AND HIJIKI SEA
veggies are rich in fiber and essential minerals, and tahini — a sesame seed paste — is rich in calcium.

½ ounce wakame seaweed, cut into small pieces

¼ ounce hijiki

½ teaspoon tahini

3 tablespoons lemon juice

1 tablespoon sesame oil

1 teaspoon grated ginger

1 tablespoon miso

¾ cup water

1 teaspoon agave, brown rice syrup, *or* local honey for sweetness *(optional)*

1 teaspoon sesame seeds for garnish

1) Soak the seaweed and hijiki in warm water for 5 minutes. Drain out the excess water and set aside.

2) In a medium bowl, combine the tahini, lemon juice, sesame oil, ginger, miso, water, and sweetener (if using). Stir until smooth.

3) Toss the seaweed with the dressing and marinate for 30 minutes. Garnish with the sesame seeds and serve.

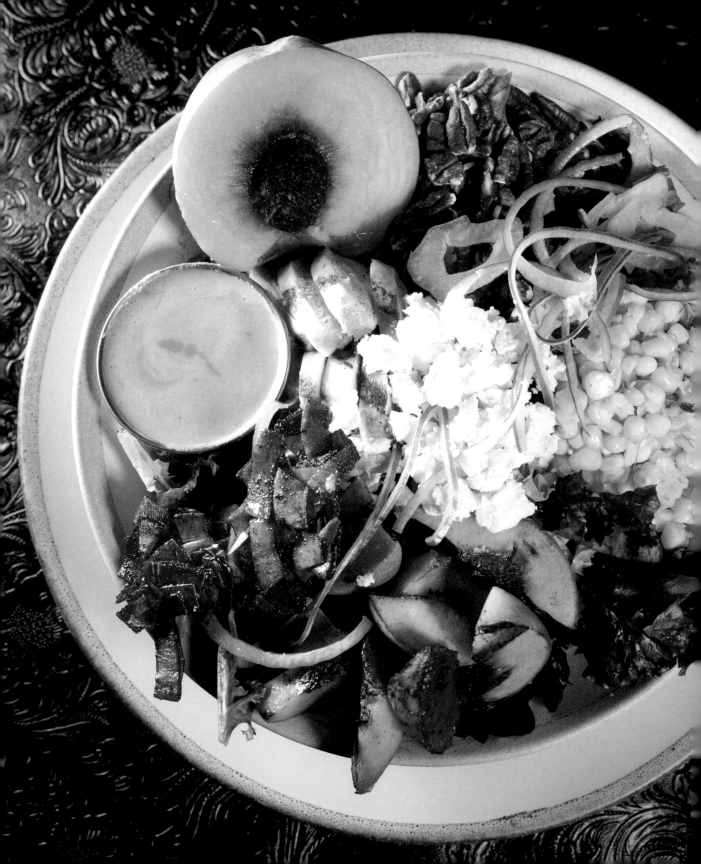

Grilled Peach Salad with Basil Chicken & Peach Cider Honey Dressing

Makes 5 servings

NOT ONLY ARE PEACHES DELISH, BUT THEY ARE ALSO STONE FRUITS, WHICH ARE supa-dupa cancer preventative, as is the vitamin K2 in dark-meat chicken. Once peaches start finding their way to Pinewood in the early summertime, we make this salad. If you don't eat meat, skip the chicken entirely and substitute with vegan options for a straight-up tasty peach salad.

FOR THE DRESSING:

⅓ cup extra-virgin olive oil

3 tablespoons apple cider vinegar

1 tablespoon local honey*

1 teaspoon Dijon mustard

1 peach, pitted and chopped

Sea salt *(to taste)*

Freshly ground black pepper *(to taste)*

Substitutions:

*If avoiding honey, replace with an equivalent amount of stevia *(see page 51).*

FOR THE CHICKEN:

2 boneless, skinless chicken breasts *or* thighs

3 tablespoons extra-virgin olive oil, plus more for the skillet

⅓ cup slightly packed, chopped fresh basil

2 cloves garlic, minced

1 tablespoon fresh lemon juice

½ teaspoon sea salt

½ teaspoon black pepper

FOR THE SALAD:

1 pound (about 3 medium) peaches, pits removed and sliced

2 cups mixed greens with arugula

2 ears corn, husked and kernels cut from cob *(optional)*

½ cup toasted, chopped pecans

½ small red onion, sliced thin *(about ¾ cup) (rinse with water to remove the harsh bite)*

¼ cup Coconut Bacon* *(see recipe page 157)*

4 ounces goat cheese *or* almond milk ricotta, crumbled

Substitutions:

*If you like pork *or* turkey bacon, feel free to use it instead.

TO MAKE THE DRESSING:

Place all the dressing ingredients in a blender or food processor and blend until creamy and smooth. Store in the refrigerator until ready to use; stir again before pouring over the salad.

TO MAKE THE CHICKEN:

1) Place the chicken between two pieces of parchment paper and pound the thicker parts of the chicken to an even thickness with a meat mallet. Transfer the chicken to a glass storage container.

2) In a small mixing bowl, whisk together the olive oil, basil, garlic, and lemon juice and season with the sea salt and pepper. Using the back of a spoon, press the basil against the sides and bottom of the bowl to help extract the flavor from the basil. Pour the basil marinade mixture over the chicken and evenly distribute the basil over the chicken. Put a lid on the container and refrigerate for 2 to 5 hours.

3) Heat a medium skillet and add the olive oil. Cook the chicken in the marinade for about 5 minutes per side or until the chicken is completely cooked. When the chicken is done, transfer it to a cutting board and let it rest for 10 minutes; slice into strips or dice into cubes.

TO MAKE THE SALAD:

1) Place the peach halves on a hot grill pan and cook for about 5 minutes max. The peaches will soften and the sugar will release, creating a sweet caramelized topping.

2) In a large salad bowl, gently toss together the peaches, greens, corn (if using), pecans, onions, grilled chicken, and bacon. Sprinkle the cheese over the top and drizzle with the dressing. Serve immediately.

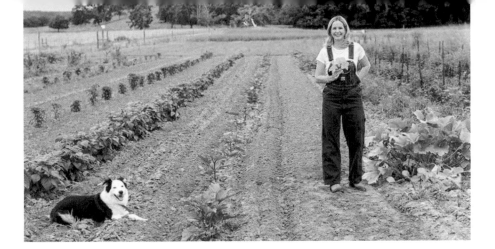

I Love Me Some Soup

What can I say? I love soup. Back when I was super sick, I struggled to digest most foods. Soup was easy to make and smooth going down. I love nuts, and pureeing them in my soups enabled me to reap their health benefits even with weak digestion. In Pinewood Kitchen, we view soups as a community development project, tweaking them a little each time we make them. The flavors of each batch can vary, depending on the produce and if it's bitter or sweet, which is dependent on the soil and weather. Play with the ingredients when you make these soups, adding more spices if you like. Feel free to add a healthy bouillon to any of your soups. Better Than Bouillon is a good organic brand. If you have a reaction to yeast, then skip the bouillon.

An important note about the soups to follow: They each include a serving of miso. Miso is great for your gut health. Traditionally, miso is made from fermented soybeans. In Pinewood, I use organic soy-free miso paste made from chickpeas because it's inclusive for soy-free folks. Whether you use soy-based or soy-free miso, just make sure that your miso is gluten free and organic. Miso Masters is a good gluten-free and organic brand. DO NOT bring soup to a boil with miso in it or you will kill the live cultures. When using miso in soups, either add a portion of diluted miso to each bowl just before serving, or add it to the blender when blending your soup. If you plan to return the soup to the pot from the blender to heat it up, hold off on the miso. Just before ladling out the portions, dilute the miso in some broth or water and add it directly to the soup pot. Your gut will thank you for it!

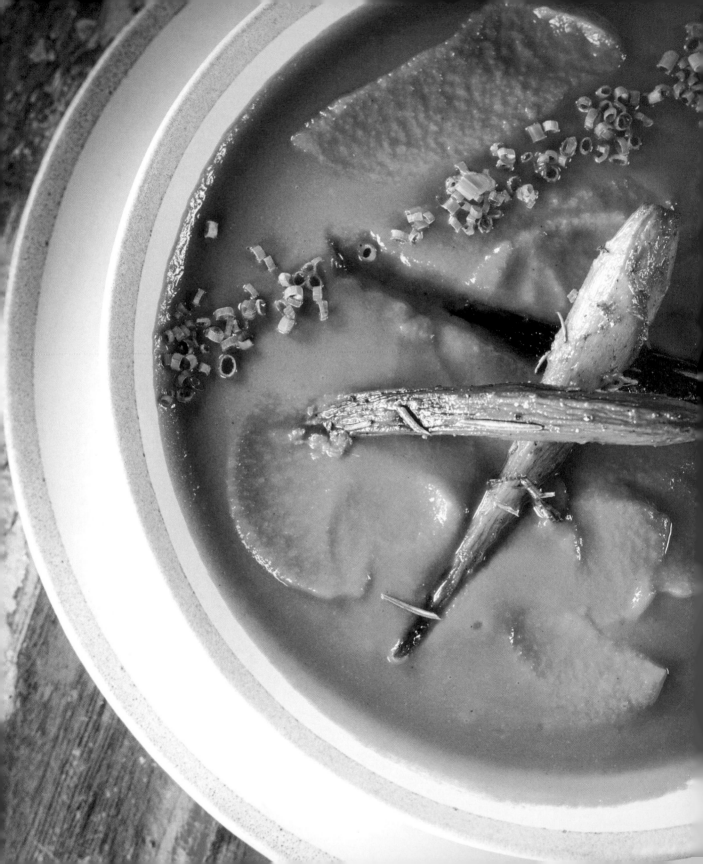

Carrot Ginger Soup

Makes 4 to 6 servings

I'M OBSESSED WITH THIS carrot soup. Sometimes all I'll have in the fridge is a bag of carrots, and that's when I make this soup happen. Carrots are great for the gut, and they are loaded with vitamin C. Granny Smith, Little Queens, or Red Delicious apples are loaded with polyphenols—they boost digestion and brain health and are believed to aid in preventing cancer. Any one of those varieties is great for this soup. The ginger is a digestive aid, as it promotes circulation. With such a powerful combination of ingredients, this soup is a soother and an immunity booster all in one bowl.

3 tablespoons extra-virgin olive oil *or* ghee

1 large white onion, diced

3 cloves garlic, minced

2 tablespoons grated fresh ginger

1½ pounds carrots

1 apple, chopped and skin on

4 cups Chicken Bone Broth *(page 120) or* Vegetable Broth *(page 121)*

2 cups water

¼ cup raw cashews

¾ cup full-fat coconut milk

1 tablespoon miso

Sea salt *(to taste)*

Freshly ground black pepper *(to taste)*

1) In a large saucepan over medium heat, heat the oil or ghee. Add the onion and sweat until soft. Add the garlic and ginger, and cook for about 3 minutes.

2) Add the carrots, apple, broth, water, and cashews. Bring to a boil and then simmer, covered, for 20 minutes. Allow to cool.

3) Transfer to a blender or food processor. Add the coconut milk and miso paste. Blend until smooth. Season with salt and pepper, to taste. Serve warm.

IT'S CLASSIC COMFORT FOOD RIGHT HERE WITH A LITTLE BIT OF A TWIST.

This soup is on the regular rotation in Pinewood Kitchen and we sell out every time. When my kids are sick or I'm feeling down, this soup brings me back around. I make this with leftover grains and roasted chicken. You can skip the chicken and add in extra carrots and mushrooms to keep it meat free.

Immune-Boosting Chicken and Quinoa Soup

Makes 4 to 6 servings

1 tablespoon extra-virgin olive oil *or* ghee

1 medium onion, chopped

3 cloves garlic, minced

3 medium carrots, chopped in small rounds

2 celery ribs, cut in ½-inch slices

1 cup chopped shiitake mushrooms

1 large bay leaf

4 cups Chicken Bone Broth *(page 120) or* Vegetable Broth *(page 121)*

2 cups water

2 cups shredded cooked chicken*

Sea salt *(to taste)*

Freshly ground black pepper *(to taste)*

Zest of 1 lemon

1 cup cooked quinoa *or* short-grain brown rice or black rice

2 tablespoons miso diluted in ¼ cup water *or* broth

3 tablespoons hijiki sea vegetable, hydrated in 1 cup water

4 to 6 lemon wedges

Several sprigs of fresh parsley or 2 tablespoons chopped parsley to garnish

Substitutions:

*If meat free, omit the chicken.

1) In a large saucepan over medium heat, heat the olive oil or ghee. Add the onion, garlic, carrots, celery, mushrooms, and bay leaf. Cook for about 6 minutes, stirring occasionally, until the vegetables have softened but not browned.

2) Add the broth and water and bring to a boil.

3) Add the chicken; season with salt and pepper, to taste, and add the lemon zest. Stir in the cooked quinoa.

4) Add the diluted miso paste to the soup, and stir. Hydrate the hijiki in 1 cup of water and rinse. Add the hijiki to the soup just before serving. Squeeze a lemon wedge over each serving to brighten up the soup and garnish with parsley.

Minty White Bean & Ham Hock Soup

Makes 4 to 6 servings

THIS RECIPE IS SO Southern and classic that it's practically part of the floorboards in Pinewood. Classic Southern cooking uses all parts of the hog, from the rooter to the tooter. Ham hocks add flavor and are usually paired with beans or greens. I always add a soy-free miso paste to my beans before serving because the miso is a probiotic. White beans are prebiotic, and that means they nourish our probiotics so they can grow and strengthen our overall health.

2 teaspoons extra-virgin olive oil

1 large onion, coarsely chopped

2 stalks celery, trimmed and coarsely chopped

1 medium carrot, coarsely chopped

2 cloves garlic, crushed

1 organic ham hock *(about 2 pounds)*

8 cups water *or* Vegetable Broth *(page 121)*

3 cups cooked white navy beans*

1 heaping tablespoon miso

Splash tamari *or* coconut aminos

Sea salt *(to taste)*

Freshly ground black pepper *(to taste)*

⅓ cup finely chopped fresh mint

*Prepare your beans according to "The Rules of Beans" on page 61.

1) Heat the oil in a large saucepan over medium heat; cook the onion, celery, carrot, and garlic, stirring until the vegetables soften.

2) Add the ham hock and the water or broth; bring to a boil. Reduce the heat and simmer, covered, for 1 hour 30 minutes. Uncover, and simmer for 30 minutes.

3) Remove the ham hock from the soup; when cool enough to handle, remove the meat from the bone and shred coarsely. Discard the skin, fat, and bone.

4) Add the beans to the soup and simmer uncovered, for 5 minutes, or until the beans are tender. Cool the soup for 10 minutes.

5) Using an immersion blender, blend the soup in the pan until it's almost smooth. Add the miso and tamari or coconut aminos. Return the ham meat to the soup with the meat juice and stir. Season with salt and pepper to taste. Top the soup with the mint and serve.

Roasted Squash & Sweet Potato Soup

Makes 4 servings

ONE OF THE THINGS

I love about this soup is that it can be made in parts. Some mornings I wake up super early with the girls, prepare breakfast, and then get all the veggies in the oven. When I come home from work, I turn the veggies into a soup. Sometimes in Pinewood, I offer something to my gluten-free customers that they are not accustomed to being offered: gluten-free croutons. I don't make them often, but when I do, they really spruce up the soup.

1 whole butternut squash, unpeeled, halved lengthwise, seeds removed

1 small sweet potato, peeled and coarsely chopped

1 medium yellow onion, peeled and quartered

4 to 5 cloves unpeeled garlic plus 1 extra clove garlic, peeled and crushed

2 tablespoons extra-virgin olive oil, divided

4 slices whole-grain gluten-free bread, cut into ¾-inch pieces

½ teaspoon crushed red pepper flakes

1 cup Vegetable Broth *(page 121) or* Beef *or* Chicken Bone Broth *(page 120)*

2 tablespoons miso

1 cup water

¼ cup Cashew Sour Cream *(page 213) or* almond milk ricotta

2 tablespoons chopped chives

2 tablespoons micro herbs *(aka micro greens)*

1) Preheat the oven to 425°F.

2) Place the squash, sweet potato, onion, and unpeeled garlic on a large baking tray; drizzle with 1 tablespoon of the oil. Bake for 45 minutes or until golden and tender. Cool for 10 minutes.

3) Meanwhile, on a baking sheet lined with parchment paper, toss the bread with the remaining oil, crushed garlic, and red pepper flakes. Bake for 15 minutes or until crisp.

4) Scoop the flesh from the squash into a blender or food processor. Discard the skins from the roasted garlic and add the garlic to the blender along with the remaining roasted vegetables.

5) Add the broth, miso, and water to the blender or food processor and blend until smooth and creamy. Divide the soup into four bowls; top evenly with the cashew sour cream, chopped chives, and micro herbs. Sprinkle each bowl with equal portions of croutons, and serve.

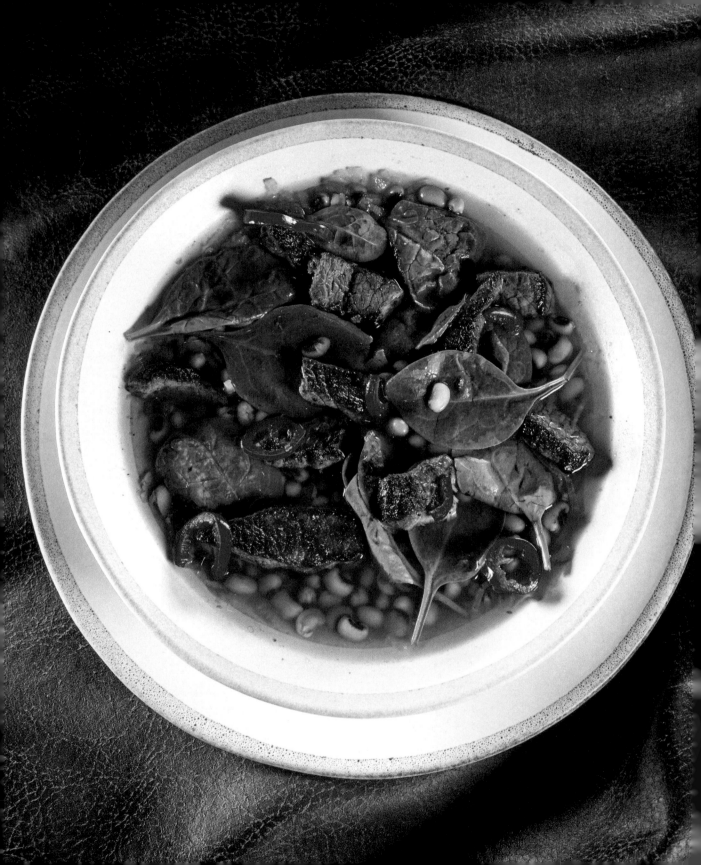

Purple-Hull Pea & Spinach Beef Soup

Makes 4 servings

PURPLE-HULL

peas are also known as cowpeas, or crowder peas. They are in the same family as black-eyed peas. On our farm, their season is August, so when we harvest them, we put them up (freeze them) or can them so that we can enjoy them for the rest of the year.

1 cup dried purple-hull peas *or* black-eyed peas

1 tablespoon extra-virgin olive oil

1 medium onion, chopped finely

1 clove garlic, crushed

10 cups Beef Bone Broth *(page 120)*

¼ cup dry red wine

2 tablespoons tomato paste

1 pound beef skirt steak

8 ounces trimmed fresh spinach, coarsely chopped

Sea salt *(to taste)*

Freshly ground black pepper *(to taste)*

2 tablespoons miso diluted in ¼ cup water *or* broth

1) Soak the peas overnight in a medium bowl filled with water. Drain, and rinse the peas well under cold water. Allow the excess water to drain out.

2) In a large saucepan over medium heat, heat the oil. Add the onion and garlic, stirring constantly until the onion softens.

3) Add the broth, wine, tomato paste, and whole skirt steak to the pan; bring to a boil. Reduce the heat to a simmer and cover. Cook for 40 minutes and remove the lid. Simmer uncovered for 30 more minutes.

4) Remove the skirt steak from the saucepan and set aside.

5) Add the peas to the saucepan and bring to a boil. Reduce the heat and simmer, uncovered, until the peas are tender, about 12 minutes.

6) When the beef is cool enough to handle, slice away and discard the fat and sinew (the tough, fibrous ligaments and tissue). Chop the meat coarsely and return it to the saucepan.

7) Add the spinach. Simmer, uncovered, until the soup is hot. Season with sea salt and black pepper, to taste, and stir in the diluted miso paste. Serve hot.

Hearty Winter Soup

Makes 4 servings

I CRAVE ROOT VEGGIES, BUT THEY WEREN'T ALWAYS PART OF MY DIET.
I was missing out on an entire group of prebiotic-rich food, and I believe that's partly why I got so sick. Not only are root veggies delicious and nutritious, but they also help us stay grounded in the winter. In fact, they're so in sync with the seasons that they offer our bodies the perfect nourishment.

2 tablespoons extra-virgin olive oil, divided

2 pounds grass-fed and finished beef stew meat*

2 shallots, halved

2 cloves garlic, crushed

2 small parsnips, coarsely chopped

2 small turnips, coarsely chopped

2 medium rutabagas, coarsely chopped

10 ounces butternut squash, coarsely chopped

1 cup organic sake *(optional)*

3 cups Beef Bone Broth *(page 120) or* Vegetable Broth *(page 121)*

3 cups water

1 tablespoon tomato paste

4 sprigs fresh thyme

Sea salt *(to taste)*

Freshly ground black pepper *(to taste)*

2 tablespoons miso diluted in ¼ cup water *or* broth

Substitutions:

*If meat free, replace with 2 cups of cooked chickpeas.

1) In a large saucepan over medium-high heat, heat 1 tablespoon of the oil. Cook the beef in batches, until browned. Remove from the pan. (If replacing beef with chickpeas, skip this step, and add them with the veggies.)

2) Turn the heat to medium and heat the remaining oil. Add the shallots and the garlic, stirring constantly, until the shallots soften.

3) Return the beef to the saucepan. Add the parsnips, turnips, rutabagas, and butternut squash. Stir.

4) Add the sake (if using), broth, water, tomato paste, and thyme; bring to a boil. Reduce the heat and simmer, stirring occasionally, for 1 hour and 30 minutes or until the beef is tender.

5) Season with sea salt and pepper, to taste. Add the diluted miso paste, stir to incorporate, and serve.

Italian Sausage & Kale Soup

Makes 4 to 6 servings

IN PINEWOOD, WE MAKE THIS SOUP AT LEAST ONCE A WEEK. ANY VARIETY OF KALE will work, and Aleppo pepper is super flavorful and adds a mild bit of heat. To make this recipe more inclusive, sauté the sausage in a separate pan with garlic, a dash of Aleppo pepper, and ¼ cup chopped onion. Set this aside and add it to the soup as you serve it; this way, if one of your guests is vegan or has the alpha-gal allergy (a meat allergy), they can also enjoy the soup.

1 tablespoon extra-virgin olive oil

1 pound ground Italian organic pork sausage*

1 medium onion, chopped

3 garlic cloves, minced

1 (28-ounce) can crushed San Marzano tomatoes *or* 2 cups fresh heirloom tomatoes

3 cups finely chopped carrots

1 teaspoon dried oregano

¼ teaspoon sea salt

⅛ teaspoon Aleppo pepper

5 cups Chicken Bone Broth *(page 120)* or Vegetable Broth *(page 121)*

2 cups cooked Northern beans** *or* 2 *(15.5-ounce)* cans great Northern beans, rinsed and drained

6 cups chopped fresh kale, ribs removed

2 tablespoons miso diluted in ¼ cup water *or* broth

Substitutions:

* If meat free, omit the sausage.

** Prepare your beans according to "The Rules of Beans" on page 61.

1) In a large saucepan, brown the sausage in olive oil and crumble. Transfer the sausage to a bowl and set aside. Pour off the extra fat. Add the onion and garlic and sauté until soft, about 5 minutes.

2) Add the tomatoes, carrots, oregano, sea salt, Aleppo pepper, broth, and sausage, and bring to a low boil, and cook for 15 minutes. Add the beans and kale, cover, and simmer for 15 more minutes. Add the diluted miso before serving.

BLACK BEANS ARE A GREAT PREBIOTIC FOOD. WITH OR WITHOUT THE chicken, this chili is simply yummy — perfect comfort food for a cold winter day!

Black Bean Chicken Chili

Makes 4 to 6 servings

¾ pound organic boneless, skinless chicken breasts, cut into 1¼-inch pieces*

¼ teaspoon sea salt

¼ teaspoon black pepper

2 tablespoons extra-virgin olive oil, divided

1 medium onion, chopped

1 jalapeño pepper, seeded and chopped

4 cloves garlic, minced

2 teaspoons dried oregano

1 teaspoon ground cumin

2 cups cooked black beans** *or* 2 *(15-ounce)* cans black beans, rinsed and drained, divided

2 small sweet potatoes, peeled and cubed

2½ cups Chicken Bone Broth *(page 120)*, divided

2 tablespoons miso diluted in ¼ cup water *or* broth

Optional Toppings:

Avocado slices

Cherry tomatoes, quartered

Cashew Sour Cream *(page 213)*

Coconut Sour Cream *(page 214)*

Chopped fresh cilantro

Substitutions:

*If meat free, replace the chicken with 2 sweet potatoes, cubed, *or* 3 carrots, chopped.

**Prepare your beans according to "The Rules of Beans" on page 61.

STOVETOP DIRECTIONS:

1) Toss the chicken with sea salt and black pepper. In a large saucepan over medium heat, heat 1 tablespoon of the oil. Brown the chicken on all sides and remove from the saucepan and set aside.

2) Add the remaining oil and the onion to the saucepan. Sauté the onion until tender. Add the jalapeño, garlic, oregano, and cumin; stir over heat for 2 more minutes.

3) Return the chicken to the saucepan, and add the beans, sweet potatoes, and the broth. Cook for 20 minutes uncovered.

4) Add the diluted miso and stir. Serve with optional toppings, if desired.

Coconut–Sweet Potato–Lentil Soup

Makes 4 to 6 servings

THIS IS THE FIRST recipe I created on my own. Now it's one of our top-requested soups in Pinewood Kitchen. The combo of sweet potatoes and orange lentils are an easy, soft, digestible fiber that gives me just what my intestines need. Slightly sweet and savory, this is a recipe that everyone loves—especially little kids. If your digestion is weak, puree the soup at the end of cooking and enjoy.

1 cup orange lentils *or* green lentils

3-inch piece kombu

4 cups Vegetable Broth *(page 121) or* Chicken *or* Beef Bone Broth *(page 120)*

2 cups water

2 tablespoons sesame oil

2 tablespoons grated fresh ginger

1 tablespoon fresh *or* dried turmeric

½ onion, diced

3 medium sweet potatoes, peeled and diced

1 clove garlic, crushed

2 tablespoons mild curry powder *(optional)*

2 tablespoons tamari *or* coconut aminos

2 tablespoons miso diluted in 1 cup coconut milk

⅛ cup chopped cilantro for garnish *(optional)*

1) In a bowl, soak the lentils in water with the kombu for 30 minutes. Rinse the lentils and kombu. Chop the kombu into small pieces.

2) In a large saucepan, combine the lentils, kombu pieces, broth, and water. Bring to a boil and skim off the foam that rises to the top. Continue to boil for 10 minutes. Lower the heat to medium-low.

3) Add the sesame oil, ginger, turmeric, onion, and sweet potatoes. Add the garlic and curry powder (if using). Lower the heat to simmer, cover, and cook slowly for an hour so that all the flavors meld together. If short on time, keep the heat on medium and cook for 40 minutes.

4) Once the sweet potatoes are soft, add the tamari or coconut aminos and miso. Serve each portion with chopped cilantro, if desired.

Mushroom Soup

Makes 4 servings

EACH TIME I MAKE this soup, I rotate my mushrooms, using whatever I have in the fridge or whatever I haven't eaten in a while. I also like to add a splash of coconut aminos or tamari for a dose of fermented goodness and prebiotic magic.

4 tablespoons extra-virgin olive oil, grass-fed butter, *or* ghee

1 large onion, coarsely chopped

6½ ounces crimini brown mushrooms, thinly sliced

1 pound white, button, *or* portobello mushrooms, thinly sliced

2 cloves garlic, crushed

1 teaspoon coarsely chopped fresh thyme leaves

4 cups Vegetable Broth *(page 121)*

2 cups water

3 ounces baby spinach leaves

2 tablespoons miso diluted in ¼ cup water *or* broth

2 tablespoons coconut aminos *or* tamari

Sea salt *(to taste)*

Freshly ground black pepper *(to taste)*

4 sprigs fresh thyme *(for garnish)*

1) In a large saucepan over medium heat, heat the oil, butter, or ghee. Add the onion and cook, stirring constantly, for 5 minutes, or until the onion is soft but not browned.

2) Increase the heat to high. Add the mushrooms and cook, stirring constantly, for 5 minutes, or until the mushrooms are well browned. Stir in the garlic and thyme, and cook until fragrant.

3) Add the broth and the water. Stir, lower the heat to simmer, and cover. Cook for 15 minutes or until the mushrooms are tender.

4) Add the spinach and stir until wilted. Add the diluted miso paste and coconut aminos or tamari and season with sea salt and pepper, to taste.

5) Divide the soup into four bowls, and top each with a sprig of thyme. Serve hot.

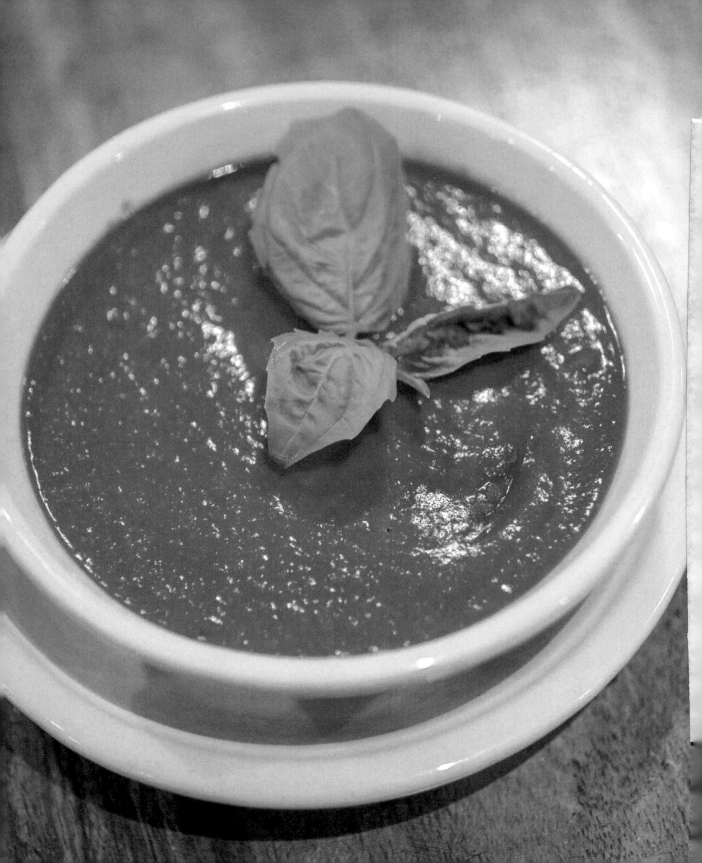

Dat's Ma Tomato Soup

Makes 4 servings

WHEN I THINK OF a soup that gives me a comforting pick-me-up, I think of tomato soup. When fighting a cold or preventing one, I make this yummy recipe. It's got protein, probiotics, and lycopene. I like to top it with fresh basil. Instead of serving this with a classic grilled cheese, we whip up delicious polenta fingers (page 115) and serve them alongside this soup.

2 tablespoons extra-virgin olive oil

1 small white onion, peeled and thinly sliced

3 cloves garlic, peeled and minced

1 *(28-ounce)* can whole peeled tomatoes *(San Marzano tomatoes are the best. In Pinewood, we use our own canned tomatoes from the farm.)*

½ cup Vegetable Broth *(page 121)*

½ cup raw unsalted cashews*

1 tablespoon nutritional yeast**

2 to 3 teaspoons coconut sugar *(optional)*

1 tablespoon chopped basil

¼ teaspoon red pepper flakes *(optional)*

1 heaping tablespoon miso

Sea salt *(to taste)*

Freshly ground pepper *(to taste)*

Substitutions:

*If nut free, replace with ½ cup chickpeas *or* 2 medium potatoes, chopped, *or* ½ head of cauliflower, chopped).

**If yeast free, omit the nutritional yeast.

1) In a large pot over medium heat, heat the olive oil. Add the onions and garlic, and sauté, stirring frequently, for 5 minutes, or until the onions are translucent and fragrant.

2) Add the tomatoes in their juices, broth, cashews, nutritional yeast, coconut sugar (if using), basil, and red pepper flakes (if using). With the back of a wooden spoon, break down the tomatoes as best as you can. Bring to a boil and simmer for 15 minutes. Remove from the heat and allow to cool.

3) Transfer the soup to a blender. Add the miso paste and puree until creamy. Add salt and/or pepper, to taste. Pour into individual serving bowls.

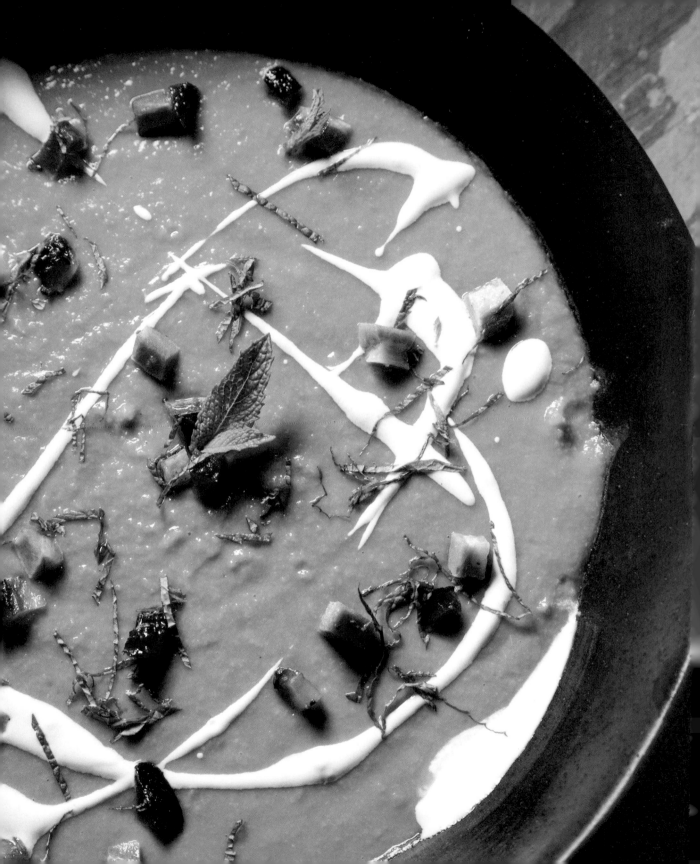

Pea, Bacon & Mint Soup

Makes 4 servings

I LOVE GREEN

peas and mint together — adding in the bacon just takes this soup to another level. Peas are a great source of protein and fiber, and leeks are loaded with prebiotic goodness. Adding in pistachios doubles this soup's prebiotic punch.

1 tablespoon extra-virgin olive oil

8 ounces pork or turkey bacon, coarsely chopped*

1 medium leek, thinly sliced

1 stalk celery, trimmed, thinly sliced

2 cloves garlic, crushed

4 cups organic frozen peas or fresh peas

4 cups Chicken Bone Broth *(page 120) or* Vegetable Broth *(page 121)*

¼ cup shelled pistachios**

2 cups water

1 cup firmly packed fresh mint

2 tablespoons miso diluted in ¼ cup water or broth

Sea salt *(to taste)*

Freshly ground black better *(to taste)*

4 sprigs mint for garnish

Substitutions:

*If meat free, replace with Coconut Bacon *(page 157)* or Tempeh Bacon *(page 158)*.

**If nut free, omit the pistachios.

1) In a large saucepan over medium heat, heat the oil. Add the bacon, leek, celery, and garlic, stirring constantly, until the onion softens and the bacon is lightly browned.

2) Add the peas, broth, pistachios, water, and mint to the saucepan; bring to a boil. Reduce the heat and simmer for 20 minutes. Cool 10 minutes and add the diluted miso paste.

3) Transfer to a blender or food processor, and blend in batches until smooth and creamy. Season with sea salt and pepper, to taste. Top with a sprig of mint and serve.

Crispy Sage, Roasted Tomato & White Bean Soup

Makes 4 servings

UNTIL GETTING WELL AND learning to cook, I only used sage in Thanksgiving dishes. But once I learned about combining flavors and sage's heart-healthy benefits, sage became my go-to herb when a recipe needed a kick. Antioxidant-rich tomatoes and sage grow together at the same time on the farm, which means they pair well on the plate. Add some miso, and now you are really supporting all healing systems.

2 pounds ripe Roma tomatoes, quartered

1 medium red onion, cut into wedges

6 cloves garlic, unpeeled

1 tablespoon local honey*

8 tablespoons extra-virgin olive oil, divided

½ cup loosely packed sage leaves

2 cups cooked white kidney beans** *or* 1 *(15.5-ounce)* can cannellini beans, rinsed and drained

2 cups water

6 cups Chicken or Beef Bone Broth *(page 120) or* Vegetable Broth *(page 121)*

2 tablespoons miso diluted in ¼ cup water *or* broth

Sea salt *(to taste)*

Freshly ground black pepper *(to taste)*

Substitutions:

*If watching sugar, omit the honey.

**Prepare your beans according to "The Rules of Beans" on page 61.

1) Preheat the oven to 400°F.

2) In a roasting pan, spread out the tomatoes, onion, and garlic. In a small bowl, mix together the honey and 4 table-spoons of the oil.

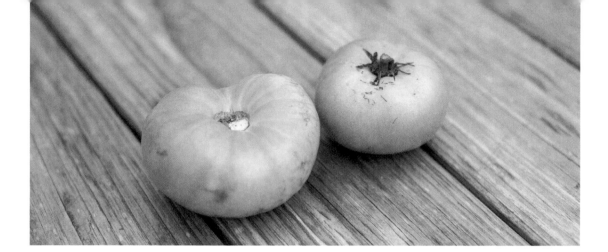

3) Pour the honey mixture over the vegetables, and toss to coat. Roast for 45 minutes or until the tomatoes are very soft and browned at the edges.

4) Meanwhile, in a small frying pan over medium heat, heat the remaining 4 tablespoons of oil. Add the sage leaves, stirring constantly, for 1½ minutes, or until the sage is crisp—be careful not to burn it. Remove the sage with a slotted spoon; drain on paper towels. Reserve the sage oil.

5) Remove the peel from the roasted garlic and discard. In a blender or food processor, combine the garlic, onion, two-thirds of the tomatoes, and two-thirds of the beans. Blend until smooth. Pour the mixture into a large saucepan. Add the water, broth, and the remaining beans; cook over medium heat, stirring occasionally until heated through. Add the diluted miso paste. Season with sea salt and black pepper, if desired, to taste.

6) Divide the soup into four bowls. Top evenly with the remaining tomatoes and crisp sage leaves; drizzle each portion with the sage oil.

Why I Love to Marry Tomatoes & Sage

Tomatoes are loaded with lycopene, a carotenoid—a natural pigment that gives some vegetables and fruits their red color. Lycopene is an antioxidant, which protects against cell damage and therefore is believed to be a major part of a cancer- and illness-preventative diet. Meanwhile, sage is an anti-inflammatory plant that has anti-hyperglycemic properties that help lower blood glucose levels—this is important for anyone who wants to prevent diabetes as well as those folks trying to keep it under control. High amounts of fats in the blood can cause high cholesterol and impact overall heart health. Sage leaf extract can help decrease the fat or bad cholesterol in the blood. Reducing these compounds allows the heart to be strong and healthy.

Cream of Celery Root Soup

Makes 8 servings

CELERIAC ROOT IS
not celery although they
are in the same family
and have a similar flavor.
Celery root is mild in
comparison to celery. It
is also loaded with trace
minerals, B vitamins,
and vitamins K and C. I
like to add a bit to my
mashed potatoes or serve
it as a mashed potato
replacement. This soup is
pure earthy goodness!

4 pounds celery root, coarsely chopped

1 medium onion, coarsely chopped

1 stalk celery, trimmed and coarsely chopped

3 cloves garlic, peeled and quartered

½ cup soaked cashews *or* blanched almonds

6 cups water

4 cups Vegetable Broth *(page 121)*

Sea salt *(to taste)*

Black pepper *(to taste)*

2 tablespoons fresh lemon juice

2 tablespoons miso diluted in ¼ cup water *or* broth

⅓ cup fresh chervil leaves *or* flat-leaf parsley

1 tablespoon extra-virgin olive oil

Fermented hot sauce or sriracha *(optional)*

1) In a large saucepan over medium heat, combine the celery root, onion, celery, garlic, cashews or almonds, water, and broth, and bring to a boil.

2) Reduce the heat to simmer and cover. Cook for 60 minutes or until tender. Remove the pan from the heat; let it stand, uncovered, for 10 minutes.

3) Transfer to a blender or food processor, and blend in batches until smooth and creamy.

4) Return the soup to the saucepan, and stir over medium heat until hot. Season with sea salt and black pepper, to taste. Stir in the lemon juice and add the diluted miso. Divide into eight portions, and sprinkle each with chervil or parsley leaves. Drizzle with oil and a swirl of fermented hot sauce or sriracha if you like things spicy.

Hot and Sour Soup with Bok Choy and Tofu

Makes 4 to 6 servings

I AM CRAZY FOR

Napa cabbage and bok choy. This is a super-quick soup to whip up, and it mixes up our traditional Southern table by using Asian flavors. I've included tofu in this recipe, but you can add leftover chicken or keep it meat free by adding extra mushrooms.

1 tablespoon dark sesame oil

4 ounces fresh shiitake mushrooms, stems finely chopped and caps thinly sliced

2 cloves garlic, minced

2 cups Vegetable Broth *(page 121)*

1 cup plus 2 tablespoons cold water, divided

2 tablespoons tamari *or* coconut aminos

1½ tablespoons rice vinegar *or* apple cider vinegar

¼ teaspoon red pepper flakes

1½ tablespoons arrowroot powder *or* kuzu root

2 cups coarsely chopped bok choy leaves *or* Napa cabbage

10 ounces extra-firm tofu, well-drained and cut into ½-inch cubes*

2 tablespoons miso diluted in ¼ cup water or broth

1 scallion, thinly sliced

Substitutions:

*If soy free, replace with 10 ounces of cooked chicken *or* omit entirely.

1) In a large saucepan over medium heat, heat the oil. Add the mushrooms and garlic; cook for 4 minutes, stirring occasionally. Add the broth, 1 cup of the water, tamari sauce or coconut aminos, vinegar, and red pepper flakes; bring to a boil. Reduce the heat to low; cook for 5 minutes.

2) In a small bowl, whisk together the remaining 2 tablespoons of water and the arrowroot or kuzu root until smooth. Stir into the soup; cook for 2 more minutes or until thickened.

3) Stir in the bok choy or cabbage; cook for 2 to 3 minutes or until the leaves are wilted. Stir in the tofu and heat through. Add the diluted miso paste. Sprinkle each serving with some of the scallions.

WHAT MOST FOLKS DON'T KNOW
is that red peppers are actually green
peppers that have been allowed to ripen
on the vine. Since they have reached
optimal fruition, they are easier to digest
than green peppers. We grow a variety
of peppers, and my favorite is a Carmen.
But if you can't find Carmens, then use
standard red peppers. These polenta
fingers are easy to make and a great thing
to prepare with leftover polenta.

Red Pepper Soup with Crispy Polenta Fingers

Serves 6

Grapeseed oil cooking spray

4 medium red bell peppers

2 cloves garlic, unpeeled

1 tablespoon olive oil

1 medium onion, chopped finely

1 teaspoon sweet paprika

3 cups water

4 cups vegetable broth

2 tablespoons miso paste

½ cup full-fat coconut milk cream

1 tablespoon finely chopped fresh chives

FRIED POLENTA

1 cup instant polenta

3½ cups water

1½ tablespoons vegan *or* grass-fed butter *or* ghee

½ cup vegan cheese *or* goat cheese

Grapeseed oil, to shallow-fry

1) Preheat the oven broiler. Quarter the peppers, discarding the seeds and the membranes. On a sheet pan sprayed with oil, roast the garlic and pepper under the hot broiler, skin-side up, until the skin blisters and blackens. Place the peppers in a covered skillet with a lid for 5 minutes; once the peppers have cooled, peel away the skin. Peel the garlic and chop it coarsely.

2) Heat the olive oil in a large saucepan over medium heat; cook the onion, stirring until softened. Add the paprika and cook, stirring, until fragrant.

3) Add the water, broth, peppers, and garlic to the pan; bring to a boil. Reduce the heat and simmer, uncovered, for 40 minutes. Cool for 10 minutes.

4) Add the miso paste and blend or process the soup, in batches, until it reaches a smooth consistency. Return the soup to the pan and add the coconut cream; stir over medium heat until hot. Season. Sprinkle the soup with the chives. Serve with polenta fingers.

TO MAKE FRIED POLENTA:

1) Cook the polenta in the water per package directions. Stir in the butter and the vegan cheese or goat cheese. Spoon the polenta into a parchment paper-lined 9-inch x 13-inch pan. Refrigerate until set.

2) Just before serving, turn out onto a cutting board; cut into 18 fingers. Heat 3–4 tablespoons of grapeseed oil in a large frying pan until hot. Fry the polenta fingers, in batches, until golden.

Black Bean Powerhouse Soup

Makes 4 to 6 servings

BLACK BEANS ARE considered super prebiotic food for Prevotella and Ruminococcus, two important anti-inflammatory bacteria. In this recipe, the bran on the brown rice is another healthy supporter of gut bacteria. Plus, the bran is loaded with health-supporting bioactives and polyphenols. This soup is perfect for those who are rebuilding their guts and react to eating beans and brown rice in whole forms. Soaking the brown rice overnight removes the phytic acid, which is believed to impair the absorption of minerals. This soup helps support the lining of the intestines, making them stronger and able to function better so they can absorb nutrients with ease.

¼ cup diced onions

2 tablespoons crushed garlic

¼ cup diced green, yellow, and red peppers plus extra for garnish

3 tablespoons extra-virgin olive oil

¼ cup dried brown rice

6 cups water

2 teaspoons ground cumin

1 teaspoon ground coriander

½ cup chopped fresh cilantro

¼ cup diced carrots

1½ cups cooked black beans* *or* 1 (15-ounce) can black beans, drained and rinsed

2 tablespoons miso

Bunch cilantro leaves for garnish

4 to 6 tablespoons Coconut Sour Cream *(page 214)*

*Prepare your beans according to "The Rules of Beans" on page 61.

1) In a large saucepan over medium heat, sauté the onions, garlic, and peppers in the olive oil until the onions are translucent, about 5 minutes. Stir in the brown rice, tossing with the onions, garlic, and bell peppers, lightly toasting the brown rice.

2) Cover with the water; add the cumin, coriander, cilantro, carrots, and black beans. Cook the soup over medium heat for 30 minutes or until the rice is soft.

3) Transfer to a blender or food processor; add the miso paste and blend until smooth and creamy.

4) Top each portion with diced peppers, cilantro leaves, and a dollop of Coconut Sour Cream.

Cream of Spinach Soup

Makes **6** servings

THIS SOUP IS A GIFT from my dear friend Señora Gina. When we lived in Sayulita, Mexico, and I could barely eat, she'd make this soup for me. Of course, once I discovered I had a major dairy allergy, I replaced the dairy with potatoes and nuts, which are super creamy when blended. Now this soup is part of our regular rotation in Pinewood.

3 tablespoons extra-virgin olive oil *or* grass-fed butter *or* ghee

1 large onion, finely chopped

2 cloves garlic, crushed

3 small purple potatoes, coarsely chopped

¾ cup blanched almond slivers *or* soaked cashews

3 cups Vegetable Broth *(page 121)* or Chicken Bone Broth *(page 120)*

4 cups water

2 cups trimmed spinach, coarsely chopped

2 tablespoons miso

Sea salt *(to taste)*

Freshly ground black pepper *(to taste)*

½ cup loosely packed, fresh flat-leaf parsley leaves

1) In a large saucepan over medium heat, heat the oil, butter, or ghee. Add the onion and garlic, stirring constantly, until the onion softens.

2) Add the potatoes, almond slivers or cashews, broth, and water; bring to a boil. Reduce the heat to simmer and cover. Cook for 15 minutes, or until the potatoes are tender. Stir in the spinach and cool for 15 minutes. Add the miso paste.

3) Transfer to a blender or food processor, and blend in batches until smooth and creamy. Return the soup to the saucepan, and stir over medium heat until hot. Season with sea salt and black pepper, to taste. Divide the soup into six soup bowls, sprinkle evenly with the parsley leaves, and serve.

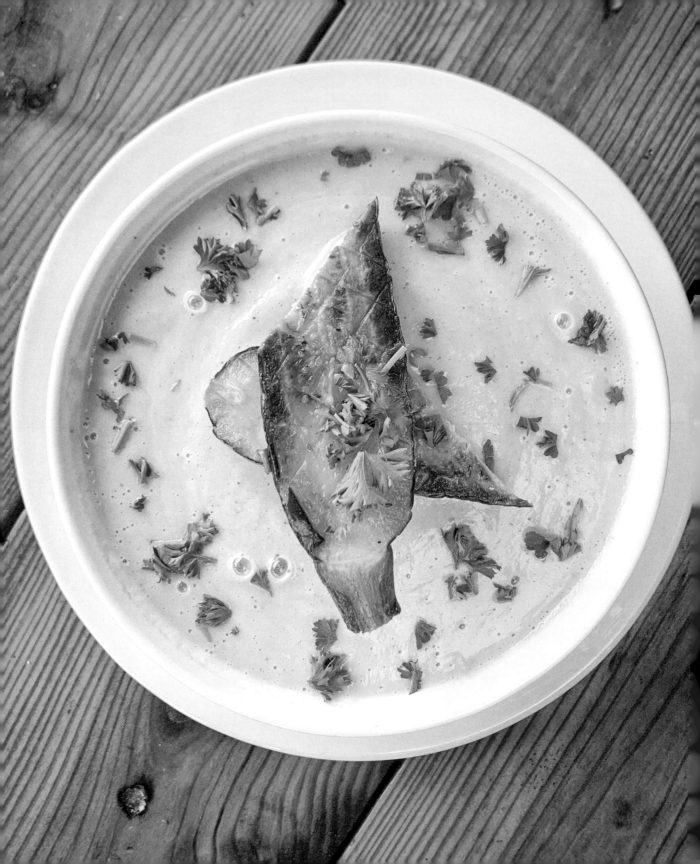

Summertime Mexican Zucchini Soup

Makes 6 servings

THIS SOUP IS A TOTAL showstopper — it's rich and creamy, and kids LOVE it. I use zucchini, but any summertime squash will work. In fact, this soup is super adaptable for any food sensitivity or health need with a little ingenuity. I love to top this soup with a dollop of Cashew Sour Cream (page 213), a drop of sriracha sauce, and a sprig of cilantro.

2 tablespoons extra-virgin olive oil *or* 1 tablespoon ghee

½ onion, chopped

3 cloves garlic, peeled and pressed *or* crushed

4 medium zucchinis with the skin on, sliced into medium rounds

3 small red potatoes with skin, halved*

¼ cup raw unsalted cashews *or* pumpkin seeds

2 tablespoons ground cumin

2 tablespoons chili powder

1 tablespoon ground coriander

¼ teaspoon cayenne pepper *(optional)*

6 cups Vegetable Broth *(page 121)* or Chicken Bone Broth *(page 120)*

4 shiitake mushrooms, stems removed and sliced

1 heaping tablespoon miso

1 cup fresh cilantro *(optional)*

Substitutions:

*If avoiding potatoes, replace with quinoa *or* just add extra zucchini.

1) Heat the oil or ghee in a large saucepan over medium heat; add the onion and cook until translucent, about 3 minutes. Stir in the garlic and zucchini. Add the potatoes, cashews or pumpkin seeds, cumin, chili powder, coriander, and cayenne pepper (if using).

2) Add the broth and mushrooms, and cover with a lid. Cook until the potatoes are tender, about 15 minutes. Cool the soup for 10 minutes.

3) Transfer to a blender or food processor. Add the miso paste and cilantro (if using), and blend until smooth and creamy. Pour the blended mixture into the saucepan, and stir over medium-high heat until hot.

Cookin' Cashews?

If you use raw cashews in a soup recipe, you do not need to soak them. By cooking them for 20 minutes or more, they will be equally as digestible as soaking them for 8 hours.

Beef Bone Broth or Chicken Bone Broth

Makes 14 cups

IN PINEWOOD, we make batches of this weekly. We run it through the canner and sell jars of it like crazy. It's the base for most of the soups I make at home and the stews in Pinewood Kitchen. You can make this with beef or chicken bones. One pound of chicken wings works great in making chicken bone broth, but any bone will do. Ham bones are great, too, so after a holiday, turn that ham bone into a broth. There is a strong belief that adding vinegar helps the collagen in the bones release.

4 pounds meaty beef bones* *or* chicken bones

2 medium yellow onions, coarsely chopped

8½ quarts water, divided

2 celery stalks, trimmed and coarsely chopped

2 medium carrots, coarsely chopped

4 cloves garlic, roughly chopped

2 teaspoons black peppercorns

3 fresh bay leaves

2 tablespoons apple cider vinegar

*Oxtail, marrowbones, or short ribs work best.

STOVETOP DIRECTIONS:

1) Preheat the oven to 350°F. Roast the bones on an oven tray for 1 hour or until browned. (If using bones from leftover roasted meat or poultry, skip this step.)

2) In a large saucepan, combine the bones and the onions with 5½ quarts of the water. Add the celery, carrots, garlic, peppercorns, and bay leaves; bring to a boil.

3) Add the vinegar and then simmer, uncovered, for 3 hours, occasionally skimming foam from the surface. Add the remaining 3 quarts of water and simmer, uncovered, for 1 hour.

4) Strain the broth through a cheesecloth-lined sieve or colander into a large heatproof bowl; discard the solids. Allow the broth to cool, cover, and refrigerate until cold. Skim and discard the surface fat before using.

Vegetable Broth

Makes 14 cups

VEGGIE BROTHS HAVE high levels of trace minerals that our digestive tracts can put to work right away. You can use just about any leftover vegetable to make a veggie broth. No veggie is wasted. I love to toss in the stems of the shiitake — it adds a tremendous depth of flavor, and all the magical healing gifts of my most favorite food.

4 medium yellow onions, coarsely chopped

2 large carrots, coarsely chopped

10 celery stalks, trimmed and coarsely chopped

2 large parsnips, coarsely chopped

2 cups mushroom stems or pieces*

6 quarts water

4 fresh bay leaves

1 teaspoon black peppercorns

*Any combination of mushrooms or single type of mushroom works great.

1) In a large saucepan over medium-low heat, add all the ingredients. Simmer, uncovered, for 1½ hours.

2) Strain the broth through a cheesecloth-lined sieve or colander into a large heatproof bowl; discard the solids. Allow the broth to cool. Cover and refrigerate until cold.

Broth Is an Individual Thing

Bone broth is believed to support the body in many ways—from strengthening the intestinal lining to boosting the immune system and infusing the body with amino acids. Veggie broths are equally powerful because they are packed with trace minerals, vitamins, prebiotic goodness, and divine tastiness.

Broth just seems to make everything better. Of course, in Mee fashion, I don't think there's just one broth for everyone. In Pinewood, we are a farm and cattle ranch. We value our livestock and are grateful for the sustenance they provide. Therefore, we use all parts of the animal. Nothing goes to waste because we don't take the livestock for granted. So bone broth is on our menu. We also serve up dishes with vegetable broth. It's an individual choice and there are many ways to enjoy the healing powers of broth.

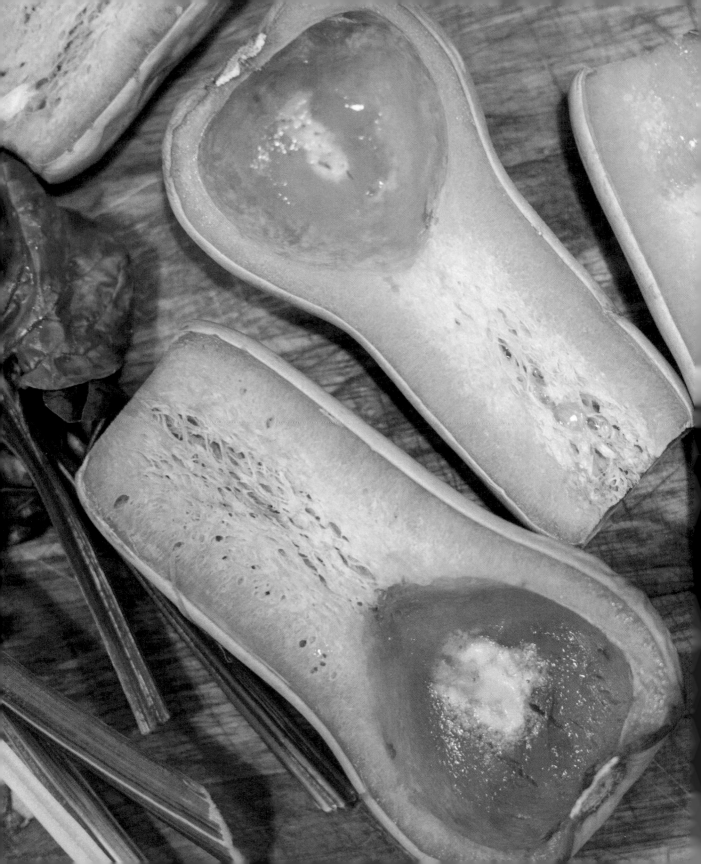

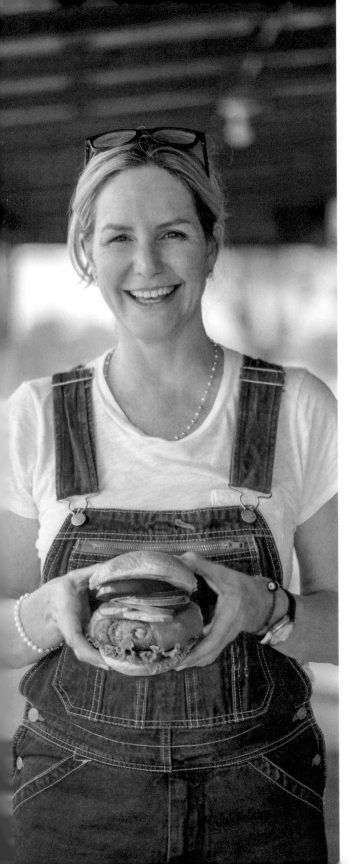

The Main Event

We run a simple menu in Pine-wood, but every weekend we focus on what's special off the farm and what meat we have in from the butcher. We raise our livestock with integrity and love. We are mindful of the environment and mob-graze our cattle, creating clean, grass-fed and finished beef. Our pork is pasture wood raised. Grass-fed animal fats contain higher proportions of omega-3 fatty acids than grain-fed animals. When we increase our consumption of omega-3 fats, our overall health benefits. I personally never eat more than 3 to 4 ounces of meat at a time and I rotate what I eat. Most of my meals are vegan because I'm always thinking about my gut health, and when I eat meat, I am sure to load my plate with an extra helping of veggies.

I LOVE BEEF STROGANOFF, AND I LOVE SHARING IT with folks who are unable to eat dairy or gluten. Mastering this dish was a big ole deal to me. Making it with ground beef is a money saver when feeding a big family, but you can easily switch it up with different cuts of meat.

Farmhouse Ground Beef Stroganoff

Makes 4 servings

2 pounds grass-fed ground beef *or* ground turkey*

1½ teaspoons sea salt

1 teaspoon black pepper

2 medium onions, chopped

2 garlic cloves, minced

1 tablespoon grass-fed butter *or* ghee**

½ pound sliced fresh shiitake mushrooms

⅓ cups Beef or Chicken Bone Broth *(page 120) or* Vegetable Broth *(page 121)*

1 tablespoon Better Than Bouillon base *(beef, chicken, or vegetarian)*

2 tablespoons tomato paste

⅓ cup 1-to-1 gluten-free flour blend***

12 ounces Cashew Sour Cream *(page 213)*

4 cups cooked gluten-free noodles *or* zucchini noodles

Substitutions:

*If meat free, replace with crumbed tempeh.

**If dairy free, replace with vegan butter.

***If grain free, replace with coconut flour.

1) Heat a large cast-iron skillet over medium-high heat. Add the ground beef or turkey, the sea salt and pepper, and cook until the meat is completely browned, about 10 minutes. Remove from the pan and set aside. Drain off the extra fat.

2) Return the pan to medium heat and add the onions; cook until translucent. Add the garlic and cook for 3 minutes more. Add the butter or ghee and the mushrooms.

3) In a glass bowl, whisk together the broth, base, tomato paste, and flour. Pour into the skillet and mix. Cook for 5 minutes, whisking to blend the flour well.

4) Add the meat back to the skillet and stir until well combined.

5) Just before serving, add the cream and mix well.

6) Serve over the noodles.

THESE SHORT RIBS ARE SO GOOD
that they'll stick to your ribs. Serve
them alongside carrots and any side
dish of your choice to indulge in
some gut-healthy comfort.

Pressure-Cooker Short Ribs

Makes 4 servings

3 pounds bone-in grass-fed and finished beef short ribs

½ teaspoon sea salt

½ teaspoon black pepper

1 tablespoon extra-virgin olive oil *or* grapeseed oil

2 large red onions, cut into ½-inch wedges

6 garlic cloves, minced

1 tablespoon tomato paste

1 cup Beef Bone Broth *(page 120)*

2 cups cabernet sauvignon wine

4 fresh thyme sprigs

1 bay leaf

4 medium carrots, cut into 1-inch pieces

4 teaspoons arrowroot powder *or* kuzu root

3 tablespoons cold water

1) Sprinkle the ribs with the sea salt and black pepper. Select the "sauté" setting on a 6-quart electric pressure cooker and adjust for high heat. Add the oil. Working in batches, brown the ribs on all sides; transfer to a plate and keep warm.

2) Add the onions to the cooker; cook and stir until tender, for 8 to 9 minutes. Add the garlic and tomato paste; cook and stir for 1 minute more. Stir in the broth, wine, thyme, and bay leaf. Bring to a boil; cook 8 to 10 minutes or until liquid is reduced by half. Add the ribs back to the cooker, partially, but not fully submerging them. Lock the lid in place; make sure the vent is closed. Select the "manual" setting; adjust the pressure to high, and set the time for 40 minutes.

3) When finished cooking, quick-release the pressure according to the manufacturer's directions. Add the carrots, bring back to full pressure, and cook for 7 minutes. Quick-release the pressure according to the directions.

4) Remove the ribs and vegetables; keep warm. Skim the fat from the cooking liquid. Discard the thyme and bay leaf. Select the "sauté" setting and adjust to high heat; bring the cooking juices to a boil. In a small bowl, mix the arrowroot powder or kuzu root with the water until smooth; stir into the juices. Return to a boil; cook and stir until thickened, 1 to 2 minutes. If desired, sprinkle with additional sea salt and black pepper.

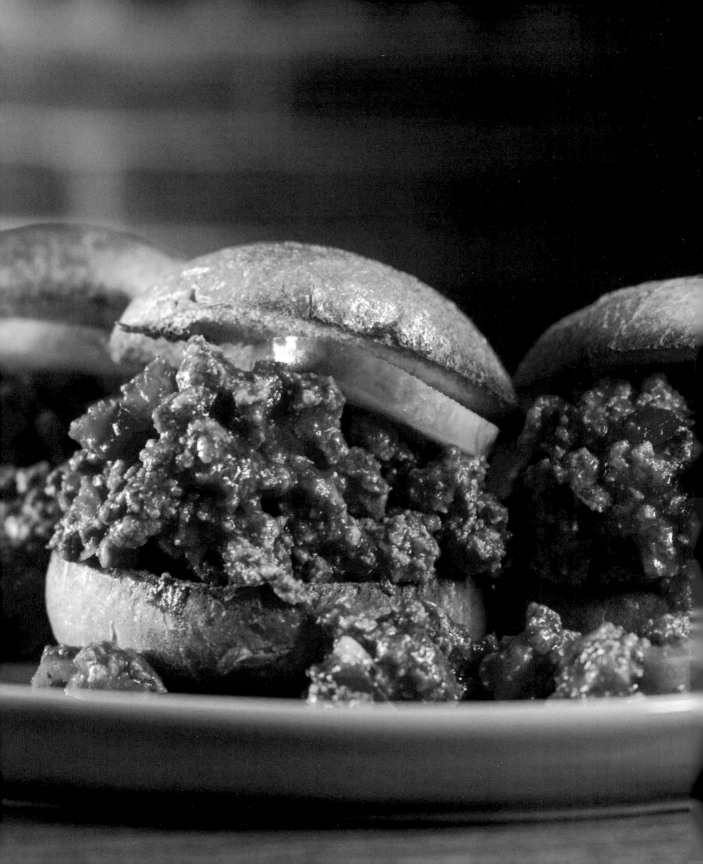

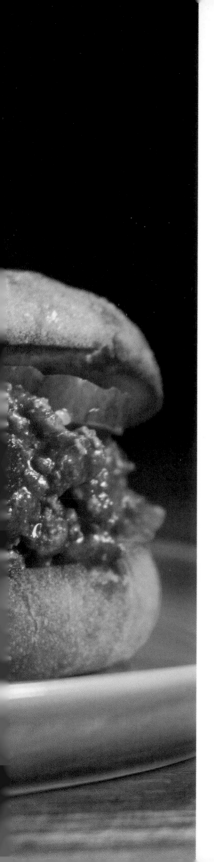

Sloppy Shawties

Makes 4 servings

I GREW UP ON sloppy joes—not out of a can but real ones my momma made with regular store-bought ketchup. I wanted to make over the classic recipe with a wellness twist, using homemade ketchup and organic grass-fed beef. Of course, I have a vegan version, too, combining leftover lentils and tempeh and following the same instructions. Serve them in lettuce cups or on gluten-free mini buns.

2 tablespoons coconut oil *or* extra-virgin olive oil

1 red bell pepper, diced

1 medium onion, diced

1 pound ground grass-fed and finished beef*

1 teaspoon sea salt

1 teaspoon crushed fresh garlic

1½ cups Dat's Ma Sup Ketchup (*page 225*)

Substitutions:

*If meat free, replace with 1 cup of cooked lentils mixed with 1 cup of cooked tempeh.

1) Warm up a large skillet over medium heat. Add the oil, pepper, and onion, and sauté for about 5 minutes or until the onion softens.

2) Add the beef, sea salt, and garlic. Stir until well combined and brown the meat completely. Add the ketchup and mix well. Simmer over low heat for 10 minutes.

Daikon Radish Is Dang Good

When I eat animal meat, I always have some grated daikon along with it. Daikon radish, which looks like a white carrot, is known to aid in digestion and flush fats from the body. It is commonly served in traditional Japanese restaurants along with fish or fried food. It has a sweet mild flavor and it makes a great condiment for burgers.

Grass-Fed Burgers Mee-ified

Makes 4 burgers

I'M **NOT GONNA LIE** — I miss a good drive-thru burger joint. But eating with celiac disease is tricky even in the nicest of restaurants. Plus, in Pinewood, we raise our own beef as ethically and naturally as possible, so now I only eat burgers from our farm. While burgers are a satisfying comfort food, I'm mindful of how often I eat meat — maybe once every six weeks tops. I serve 'em up with all the traditional fixings along with a side of collard greens or kale.

1 pound ground organic grass-fed beef

1 huge handful fresh cilantro, chopped

2 carrots, grated

1 tablespoon hydrated hijiki seaweed, minced

1 tablespoon tamari *or* coconut aminos

1 sweet potato *or* regular potato

1 zucchini, chopped small

⅛ cup finely chopped red bell pepper

¼ cup grated onion

2 cloves garlic, minced

Sea salt *(to taste)*

Freshly ground black pepper *(to taste)*

1 daikon radish, grated, for serving

1) In a large bowl, mix all the ingredients until well combined. Let the mixture sit in the fridge for several hours to blend the flavors.

2) When it's time to eat, whip out the meat mixture and make four patties. Grilling is the best, but a skillet is old-school cool. Cook the burgers to the desired doneness and serve the daikon radish on the side.

Meatball variation: This recipe also makes great meatballs. Substitute oregano for cilantro, and add some parsley, one egg, and ½ cup gluten-free breadcrumbs. If you are avoiding processed grains, use leftover quinoa or brown rice. For grain-free meatballs, use almond flour instead of breadcrumbs or just leave the breadcrumbs out.

Gluten-Free Beer Braised Brisket

Makes 4 to 6 servings

IN PINEWOOD, WE HAVE A GIANT SMOKER OUT BACK THAT BARBECUE EXPERTS
Mario and Michael run with insane style. I had zero smoking experience, and the one thing I've learned from the guys in the "pit" is that it's all about the rub and the slow cooking. This recipe is so delish that your friends are going to think you smoked it all night long.

6 cloves garlic

5 tablespoons coconut sugar

2 tablespoons Dijon mustard

2 tablespoons extra-virgin olive oil

2 teaspoons organic liquid smoke

2 teaspoons gluten-free Worcestershire sauce

1 tablespoon freshly ground black pepper

1 tablespoon smoked paprika

1 tablespoon cayenne pepper *(optional)*

¼ cup flaky sea salt, plus a touch more

1 (8- to 10-pound) untrimmed flat-cut brisket

2 large onions, sliced into thin half moons

1 bottle gluten-free beer, preferably dark

1) In a food processor, pulse the garlic until finely chopped. Add the coconut sugar, Dijon mustard, olive oil, liquid smoke, Worcestershire sauce, black pepper, paprika, cayenne pepper (if using), and sea salt. Process until smooth.

2) Rub the spice mixture all over the brisket, working into crevices. Wrap the brisket in parchment paper and then double wrap it in plastic so that the plastic doesn't touch the meat. Chill for 24 hours. Bring the meat to room temperature on the counter, about 1 hour.

3) Preheat the oven to 325°F. Spread out the onions in a large roasting pan and set the brisket on top, fat side up. Add the beer; cover with parchment paper and then cover with foil. Braise (cook slowly) until the meat is very tender, about 5 to 6 hours. Remove from the oven.

4) Heat the broiler. Return the brisket, uncovered, to the oven and broil until the top is browned and crisp, about 7 to 10 minutes.

5) Let the brisket cool slightly. Remove from the pan and shred or slice. Remove the onions with a slotted spoon and scatter over the brisket.

6) Taste and moisten with some cooking liquid; season with additional sea salt if needed.

Pinewood Grass-Fed & Finished Beef Tips

Makes 4 to 6 servings

BEEF TIPS ARE AN EASY WAY TO STRETCH A SIMPLE CUT OF MEAT. WHEN THEY ARE cooked slowly, they become super tender. Portobello mushrooms bring a nice, earthy element to the plate. You can serve this dish with mashed cauliflower or classic mashed potatoes.

3 teaspoons extra-virgin olive oil

1 pound beef top sirloin steak, cubed

½ teaspoon sea salt

¼ teaspoon black pepper

⅓ cup dry red wine*

1 small onion, halved and sliced

2 cups Beef Bone Broth *(page 120)*

½ pound sliced baby portobello mushrooms

1 tablespoon gluten-free Worcestershire sauce

3 to 4 tablespoons arrowroot powder diluted in ¼ cup cold water

*I recommend organic or biodynamic cabernet for its healing qualities.

1) In a large cast-iron skillet over medium heat, heat the olive oil. Add the beef tips, sea salt, and pepper, and cook until brown on all sides. Remove from the pan and set aside on a plate.

2) Add the red wine to the skillet to loosen up the crispy bits. Add the onion, and sauté until translucent, about 5 minutes. Add the broth, mushrooms, and Worcestershire sauce and return the beef tips to the skillet. Simmer for about 15 minutes. Stir in the diluted arrowroot. Cook and stir until the sauce is thickened, about 1 to 2 minutes.

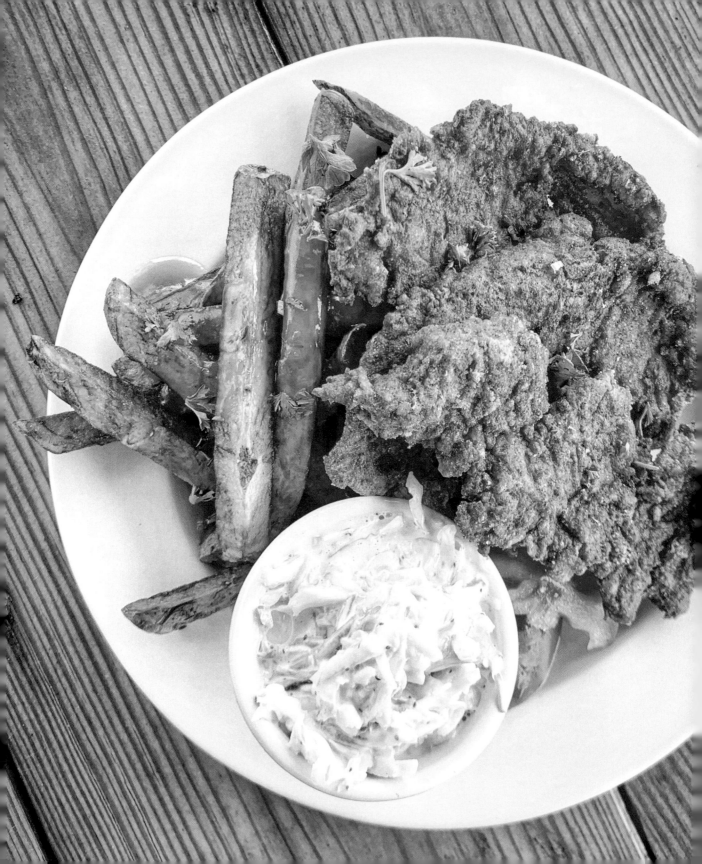

Pork Schnitzel

Makes 4 servings

DANG IT, THIS IS THE shizznitty! I swear this is one of the best things I've ever eaten. When Chef Michael made this, I had to step away from the kitchen and put the schnitzel down. I don't eat a lot of meat, and pork is something I only eat when I'm feeling tip-top, so it's a good thing we only make this once in a while. What's even better about this recipe is that it's "free" all around: gluten free, egg free, soy free, dairy free, and nut free!

4 boneless pork chops or 1½ pounds pork loin, cut into ½-inch slices

1 tablespoon smoked paprika

1 teaspoon garlic powder

1 teaspoon onion powder

½ teaspoon dry mustard

½ teaspoon white pepper

¼ teaspoon cayenne pepper

½ teaspoon sea salt

1 cup 1-to-1 gluten-free flour blend

1½ cups grapeseed oil

1) Trim the fat and silver skin off of the pork chops or pork loin. Cut through the seams on each side of a gallon freezer bag. Place two pieces of parchment paper inside the plastic bag. Place two or three pieces of the pork between the parchment, and then pound the pork thin with a meat mallet. Transfer to a large mixing bowl.

2) Add the spices to the pork, and mix well until the meat is evenly coated. Dip each piece of pork into the flour and cover both sides.

3) In a large skillet, heat the oil. Fry the pork in batches until crispy and the internal temperature has reached 165°F, about 6 minutes per side.

JUNIPER BERRIES ARE BELIEVED TO AID IN DIGESTION
by eliminating gas and bloating. Anytime I can cook with a digestive aid, I do.
Juniper berries are also believed to help stimulate the kidneys,
which is always a plus for keeping the body's filtration
system flowing with ease. Plus, they give a delicious
aromatic flavor to chicken, pork, or jackfruit,
which is often used as a meat substitute.

Juniper Berry Pan-Roasted Pork Chops

Makes 2 servings

2 cups water

½ cup sea salt

½ cup coconut sugar

1 teaspoon juniper berries

½ teaspoon black peppercorns

1 head of garlic, halved crosswise plus
2 unpeeled cloves for basting

2 large sprigs thyme

5 cups ice cubes

2 (1½-inch thick) bone-in pork chops
(about 3 pounds each chop)

2 tablespoons extra-virgin olive oil
or coconut oil

3 tablespoons grass-fed butter, ghee,
or nondairy butter

1) In a medium saucepan over medium-high heat, bring the water to a boil. To make the brine, add the sea salt, coconut sugar, juniper berries, peppercorns, halved head of garlic, and 1 of the sprigs of thyme; stir until the sea salt and sugar are dissolved.

2) Transfer the brine to a medium bowl and add the ice cubes. Stir until cool. Add the pork chop; cover and chill for at least 8 hours and up to 12 hours.

3) Preheat the oven to 450°F. Remove the pork chop from the brine; pat dry and discard the brine. Heat the oil in a large cast-iron or ovenproof skillet over medium-high. Cook the chop until beginning to brown, about 3 minutes. Turn and cook until the second side is beginning to brown, about 2 minutes. Turn the chop every 2 minutes until both sides are deep golden brown, about 10 to 12 minutes.

4) Transfer the skillet to the oven and roast the chop, turning every few minutes to prevent it from browning too quickly, until a meat thermometer inserted horizontally into the center of the meat registers 135°F, about 12 to 15 minutes. (The chop will continue to cook during basting and resting.)

5) Carefully drain the fat from the skillet and set over medium heat. Add the oil, ghee, or butter, the garlic cloves, and the remaining sprig of thyme; cook until the oil or butter is foaming. Carefully tip the skillet and, using a large spoon, baste the chop repeatedly with the buttery juices until the butter is brown and smells nutty, about 2 minutes.

6) Transfer the pork to a wire rack set inside a rimmed baking sheet and let rest, turning often to ensure the juices in the meat are evenly distributed, about 15 minutes. (Discard the marinade.) When cool, cut the meat from the bones, slice, and sprinkle with additional sea salt, if desired.

HASH IS A COMMON FOOD IN THE SOUTH.
I love to combine our farm-grown sweet potatoes
and pork tenderloin in this dish. If you're looking for
a shortcut, frozen diced sweet potatoes are perfect
for this. If you have leftovers, serve
it up for breakfast topped
with a cooked egg.

Garlic Pork and Sweet Potato Hash

Makes 4 to 6 servings

6 small sweet potatoes, skin on, cut into chunks

1½ pounds pork tenderloin, trimmed and cut into 1-inch slices

2 tablespoons Beef Bone Broth (*page 120*)

½ teaspoon sea salt

¼ teaspoon black pepper

3 tablespoons extra-virgin olive oil, coconut oil, *or* ghee

8 cloves garlic, thinly sliced

¼ cup sliced scallions

2 tablespoons local honey

2 tablespoons water

4 to 6 fresh thyme sprigs, for garnish

1) Fill a large pot of water and submerge the sweet potato chunks. Bring them to a boil, cover, and continue to boil for about 10 minutes. When the potatoes are soft, remove them from the water and allow them to cool; the skins will fall away. Once cooled, dice them and set them aside.

2) Butterfly each slice of meat by making a horizontal cut three-quarters of the way through each slice; open it and flatten slightly. Brush with 1 tablespoon of the broth and sprinkle with sea salt and black pepper.

3) In an extra-large skillet, heat the oil over medium-high heat. Add the garlic; cook and stir until just golden. Remove from the skillet. Add the meat; cook for 4 to 6 minutes or until a thermometer registers 145°F, turning once. Remove the meat from the skillet; keep warm.

4) Add the sweet potatoes to the same skillet. Cook until the potatoes are starting to crisp, stirring occasionally. Add the scallions; cook and stir for 1 minute. Spoon the hash onto serving plates; top with the meat and garlic.

5) In the same skillet, whisk together the honey, water, and remaining broth. Cook and stir until bubbly. Drizzle over the meat and top with fresh thyme sprigs.

Pork Shoulder with a Kickin' Diavolo

Makes 8 servings

PAIR THIS DISH

with any veggie side for a full meal. If you have leftovers, use them over a salad for a meal full of flavor and goodness.

1 skinless, boneless pork shoulder *or* Boston butt *(about 6 pounds)*

A few pinches sea salt

1 tablespoon black peppercorns

1 tablespoon coriander seeds

1 tablespoon crushed red pepper flakes

1 tablespoon dried oregano

1 tablespoon yellow mustard seeds

½ cup extra-virgin olive oil

6 garlic cloves, crushed

1 tablespoon finely grated lemon zest

2 teaspoons smoked paprika

1) Using the tip of a knife, lightly score the fatty side of the pork; season all over with the sea salt.

2) Coarsely grind the peppercorns, coriander seeds, red pepper flakes, oregano, and mustard seeds in a spice mill or with mortar and pestle; set the spice mixture aside.

3) In a small saucepan, heat the oil over low heat; add the garlic, stirring often, until fragrant and barely golden, about 5 minutes. Stir in the lemon zest, paprika, and reserved spice mixture. Let the marinade cool.

4) Rub the marinade all over the pork, working some marinade into the interior of the roast. Tie the pork at one-inch intervals with kitchen twine. Wrap tightly in plastic and chill for at least 8 hours.

5) Let the pork sit at room temperature for 1 hour. Preheat the oven to 375°F. Unwrap the pork, place it on a rack set inside a roasting pan, and roast until golden brown and the fat has just started to render, about 40 to 50 minutes. Reduce the oven temperature to 300°F and continue to roast until the meat is very tender, about 1½ to 2 hours. Transfer the pork to a cutting board and let it rest for 30 minutes before slicing.

Kentucky Caramel Chicken

Makes 4 servings

THERE'S NOTHING BETTER THAN COMBINING SWEET, TANGY, AND SALTY IN ONE DISH.
This is great alongside brown rice.

2 cups grapeseed oil *or* olive oil

2½ pounds skin-on, bone-in chicken thighs and drumsticks*

A few pinches sea salt

8 garlic cloves, peeled

½ cup water

⅓ cup packed light brown sugar *or* coconut sugar**

¼ cup unseasoned rice vinegar

2 ¼-inch thick slices peeled ginger

1 cup Chicken Bone Broth *(page 120) or* Vegetable Broth *(page 121)*

¼ cup tamari *or* coconut aminos

2 scallions, thinly sliced

Substitutions:

*If meat free, replace with tempeh *or* jackfruit.

**If watching sugar, replace with an equivalent amount of stevia *(page 51)*.

1) Heat the oil in a large, wide cast-iron skillet or heavy pot over medium-high heat.

2) Season the chicken all over with sea salt and, working in two batches, cook the chicken until golden brown and crisp, about 6 to 8 minutes per side; transfer the cooked chicken to a plate.

3) Add the garlic cloves to the same skillet and cook, stirring often, until golden, about 2 minutes; transfer the garlic cloves to the plate with the chicken. Pour off the fat from the pot.

4) Return the pot to medium-high heat and add the water, scraping up any brown bits. Add the sugar. Stir to dissolve, and then cook, stirring, until the mixture thickens and turns a deep amber color, about 4 minutes. Carefully add the vinegar (it may bubble up; sugar will crystalize), and then stir to dissolve the sugar. Stir in the ginger, broth, and tamari or coconut aminos.

5) Add the chicken, skin side up, along with the garlic cloves. Bring to a boil, reduce the heat, and simmer gently until the chicken is cooked through, about 20 to 25 minutes. Return the chicken and garlic to the plate.

6) Bring the cooking liquid in the pot to a boil and cook it until thick enough to coat a spoon, about 10 to 12 minutes. Return the chicken and garlic to the pot and turn to coat. Transfer to a serving plate, and sprinkle the scallions on top.

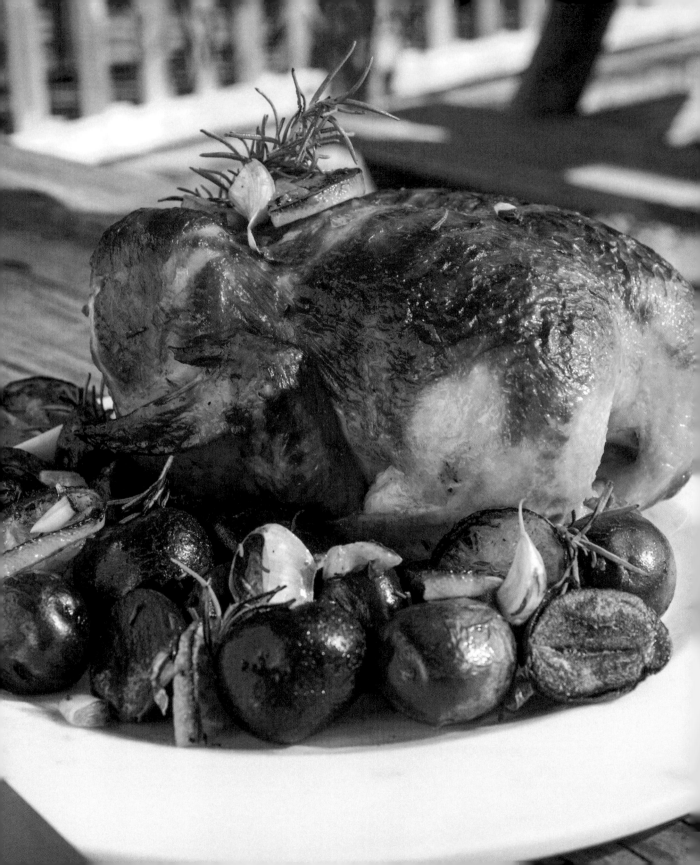

Lemon Garlic Skillet-Roasted Chicken

Makes 4 to 6 servings

LOTS OF FOLKS THINK that the white meat is healthier than dark meat. What they don't know is that dark meat contains vitamin K2, which the body requires for heart health, blood coagulation, and for calcium metabolism. I love pairing chicken with rosemary, which grows like crazy on our farm. Rosemary contains rosmarinic acid, which has many health benefits. And by roasting the chicken with purple potatoes, this dish becomes a bioactive feast!

1 lemon

2 tablespoons vegan butter *or* grass-fed butter, softened

2 sprigs fresh rosemary, finely chopped, plus 2 whole sprigs fresh rosemary

3 cloves garlic, minced, plus 3 whole cloves garlic

2 teaspoons sea salt, divided

10 small purple potatoes, cut into ¾-inch pieces

2 onions, cut into 1-inch pieces

2 tablespoons extra-virgin olive oil

½ teaspoon black pepper

1 whole organic chicken *(about 3 to 4 pounds)*

1) Preheat the oven to 400°F.

2) Grate the zest from the lemon into a small bowl. Set the lemon aside. Add the butter, chopped rosemary, minced garlic, lemon zest, and ½ teaspoon of the sea salt in a small bowl; mix well. Set aside.

3) In a medium bowl, combine the potatoes, onions, extra-virgin olive oil, 1 teaspoon of the sea salt, and black pepper, and toss to coat. Spread the potato mixture in a single layer in a large cast-iron skillet.

4) Smash the remaining 3 cloves of garlic. Cut the lemon into quarters. Season the cavity of the chicken with the remaining ½ teaspoon of the sea salt. Place the garlic, lemon quarters, and the 2 sprigs rosemary in the cavity; tie the legs together with kitchen string, if desired. Place the chicken on top of the potato mixture in the skillet; spread the butter mixture over the chicken.

5) Roast for about 1 hour or until the chicken is cooked through and the potatoes are tender. Let stand 10 minutes before carving. Sprinkle with additional sea salt and pepper, if desired.

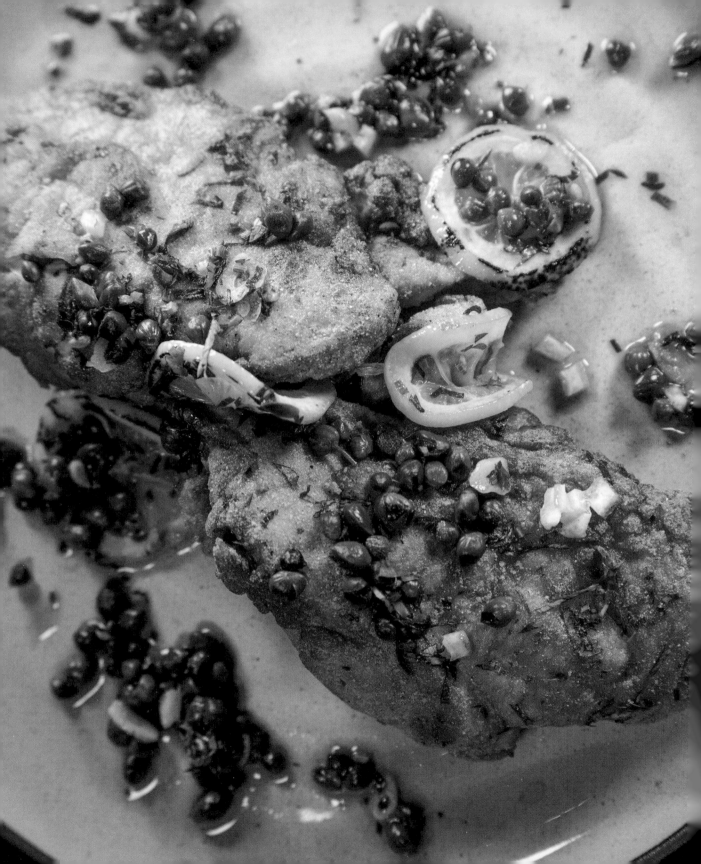

Chicken Piccata

Makes 4 servings

I ABSOLUTELY LOVE CHICKEN PICCATA; HOWEVER, FINDING IT GLUTEN FREE IN A restaurant almost never happens—unless you are dining in Pinewood Kitchen. Capers are considered a majorly important anti-inflammatory food. I love to serve this over roasted cauliflower and with zucchini noodles instead of pasta.

3 tablespoons 1-to-1 gluten-free flour blend*

½ teaspoon sea salt

¼ teaspoon black pepper

4 boneless, skinless chicken breasts**

2 teaspoons extra-virgin olive oil

1 teaspoon vegan butter, grass-fed butter, *or* ghee

2 cloves garlic, minced

¾ cup organic Chicken Bone Broth *(page 120) or* Vegetable Broth *(page 121)*

1 tablespoon lemon juice

2 tablespoons chopped fresh Italian parsley

1 tablespoon drained capers

Substitutions:

*If grain free, replace with almond flour.

**If meat free, skip the directions for cooking the chicken and replace with grilled portobello mushrooms and roasted cauliflower florets.

1) In a shallow dish, combine the flour, sea salt, and black pepper. Reserve 1 tablespoon of the mixture; set aside.

2) Pound the chicken to ½-inch thickness between sheets of parchment paper with the flat side of a meat mallet or a rolling pin. Coat the chicken with the flour mixture, shaking off excess.

3) In a large nonstick skillet over medium heat, heat the olive oil and butter. Add the chicken; cook for 4 to 5 minutes per side or until no longer pink in the center. Transfer to a serving platter; cover loosely with foil.

4) Add the garlic to the same skillet; cook and stir for 1 minute. Add the reserved 1 tablespoon of the mixture; cook and stir for 1 minute. Add the broth and lemon juice; cook 2 minutes or until thickened, stirring frequently. Stir in the parsley and capers until blended. Spoon the sauce over the chicken.

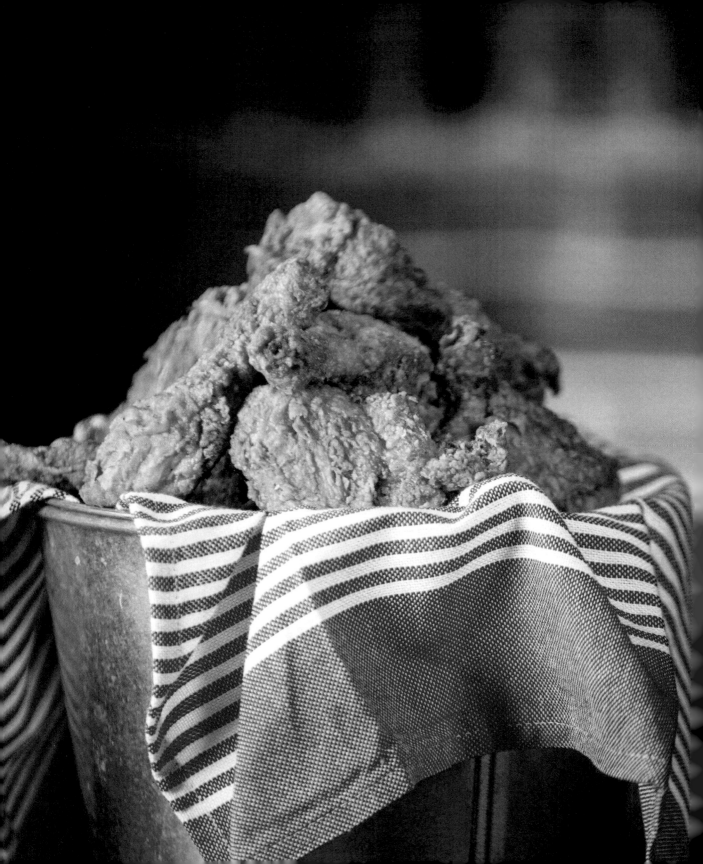

Pinewood Fried Chicken

Makes 4 servings

¼ cup sea salt, plus 1 additional teaspoon
¼ cup organic sugar *or* ¼ teaspoon stevia
3½ pounds bone-in split breasts, cut in half and fat trimmed *(drumsticks or thighs work, too)*
1 cup non-GMO cornstarch
1 egg
1 teaspoon baking powder
½ teaspoon baking soda

1 tablespoon fresh squeezed lemon juice *or* 1 tablespoon apple cider vinegar
1 cup nondairy milk
1 cup non-GMO cornmeal
1½ teaspoons garlic powder
1½ teaspoons paprika
¼ teaspoon cayenne pepper
3–4 quarts rice bran oil *or* grapeseed oil

1) To make the brine: In a quart of water, whisk the sea salt and the sugar (or stevia) together in a large bowl until they dissolve. Add the chicken, cover it, and place it in the fridge for at least an hour. Remove the chicken from the brine and pat it dry with paper towels.

2) Place ½ cup of the cornstarch in a large zipper bag. Beat the egg, baking powder, and baking soda together in a medium bowl. In a separate bowl, combine the lemon juice or apple cider vinegar with the nondairy milk. Mix together and allow to sit for 10 minutes to make "buttermilk." Stir the buttermilk into the baking powder/baking soda mixture. In a shallow dish, whisk the remaining ½ cup of cornstarch, cornmeal, garlic powder, paprika, cayenne, and 1 teaspoon salt together.

3) Place a few pieces of chicken in the bag with the cornstarch; seal the bag, and shake well to coat the chicken. Using tongs, remove the chicken pieces from the bag, shaking off the excess cornstarch. Dip the chicken in the vegan buttermilk mixture and then coat with the cornmeal mixture, pressing gently to make sure it sticks. Place the dredged chicken on a wire rack, skin-side up. Cover and let it sit for 30 minutes. This helps the coating to adhere before dropping into the fryer.

4) Add the oil to a large Dutch oven (about 2 inches of oil). Heat over medium-high heat until it reaches 350°F. Heat the oven to 200°F and make sure your oven rack is in the middle. Using tongs, carefully place the chicken in the pot, skin side down; cover, and fry, moving the chicken pieces occasionally to prevent them from sticking together. Fry until the chicken reaches a golden brown, about 7 to 12 minutes. Your oil temperature will lower with the chicken cooking in it, so make sure your oil stays between 300–325°F, using a meat thermometer. Flip your chicken pieces over, and continue to cook until the breast reaches 165°F and the drumsticks and/or thighs register at 175°F. This takes about 8 minutes.

5) Drain the chicken on paper towels or brown paper bags. Transfer the chicken to a clean wire rack set on a rimmed baking sheet and keep it warm in the oven until serving. Bring your oil back up to 350°F and continue cooking the rest of your chicken.

THIS IS OFF-THE-HOOK DELISH.

Eating dumplings in Pinewood is as old as the day is long. But cooking and eating gluten-free dumplings is what I brought to Pinewood Kitchen via my sister Nicole and Ms. Tina. The two of them whip these babies up, and on a cold winter day, we sell out.

Aunt Colie's Chicken & Dumplings

Makes 4 servings

FOR THE DUMPLINGS:

2 cups 1-to-1 gluten-free flour blend

1 teaspoon sea salt

1 cup ice water

FOR THE BROTH:

3 ribs celery, chopped

1 large onion, chopped

2 bay leaves

2 organic chicken bouillon cubes *(optional)*

½ teaspoon garlic, minced *or* crushed

6 cups water *or* broth of choice

1 whole chicken, cut into 8 pieces

1 cup fresh peas *or* frozen organic peas

1 tablespoon miso diluted in ¼ cup water *or* broth

Sea salt *(to taste)*

Freshly ground black pepper *(to taste)*

¼ cup chopped fresh parsley

TO MAKE THE DUMPLINGS:

1) In a medium mixing bowl, whisk together the flour and the salt. Pour the mixture onto a clean surface, making a well in the middle of the flour.

2) Slowly add the water until you can form a ball and then roll out the dough using a rolling pin.

3) Cut the dough into 1-inch strips or squares. Some people like dumpling-size balls, but I prefer strips.

TO MAKE THE BROTH:

1) In a large pot over medium heat, combine the celery, onion, bay leaves, bouillon (if using), and garlic. Cook until the onions soften. Cover with the water or broth.

2) Add the chicken and simmer until the chicken is tender and the thigh juices run clear, about 35 to 45 minutes. Remove the chicken from the pot and, when it's cool enough to handle, remove the skin and separate the meat from the bones. Discard the skin and bones, and shred the chicken.

3) Return the chicken to the pot. Add the peas, and simmer for 7 minutes more.

4) Drop the dumplings slowly into the simmering broth. Don't stir the broth once the dumplings have been added. Instead, gently move the liquid in the pot in a circular motion with a large spoon so the dumplings become submerged and cook evenly.

5) Cook until the dumplings float to the top and are no longer doughy, less than 5 minutes.

6) Add the diluted miso, season with salt and pepper, to taste, and top with fresh parsley.

WHO DOESN'T LOVE WINGS?
This spicy cranberry glaze is a
flavor game-changer. This recipe
is sure to become a requested
tailgating or holiday party
favorite.

Cranberry Hot Wings

Makes 4 to 6 servings

1¾ cups fresh cranberry sauce *or* 1 (*14-ounce*) can low-sugar jellied cranberry sauce

½ cup orange juice

¼ cup hot pepper sauce

2 tablespoons tamari *or* coconut aminos

2 tablespoons local honey

1 tablespoon packed brown sugar *or* coconut sugar*

1 tablespoon Dijon mustard

2 teaspoons garlic powder

1 teaspoon dried minced onion

1 garlic clove, minced

4 teaspoons arrowroot powder diluted in 2 tablespoons cold water

5 pounds chicken wings (*about 24 wings*)

1 tablespoon extra-virgin olive oil

1 teaspoon sea salt

Dash freshly ground black pepper

Substitutions:

*If watching sugar, replace with an equivalent amount of stevia (*page 51*).

1) In a small saucepan, combine the cranberry sauce, orange juice, hot pepper sauce, tamari or coconut aminos, honey, sugar, mustard, garlic powder, minced onion, and minced garlic. Whisk until well combined. Bring almost to a boil, add the diluted arrowroot, and then simmer, reducing until the sauce becomes a thick glaze. Set aside.

2) Preheat the broiler to high with an oven rack set on the bottom, farthest from the heat. Use a sharp knife to cut through the two wing joints; discard the wing tips or save to make bone broth.

3) Toss the chicken wings in olive oil until well coated and place on a baking sheet. Sprinkle with sea salt and black pepper. Broil the wings until the skin is slightly crispy and brown, about 11 to 13 minutes. Flip the wings over and cook for 7 minutes more until crisp and golden brown.

4) Remove the wings from the oven and coat with the cranberry glaze. Return to the broiler for 3 to 4 minutes.

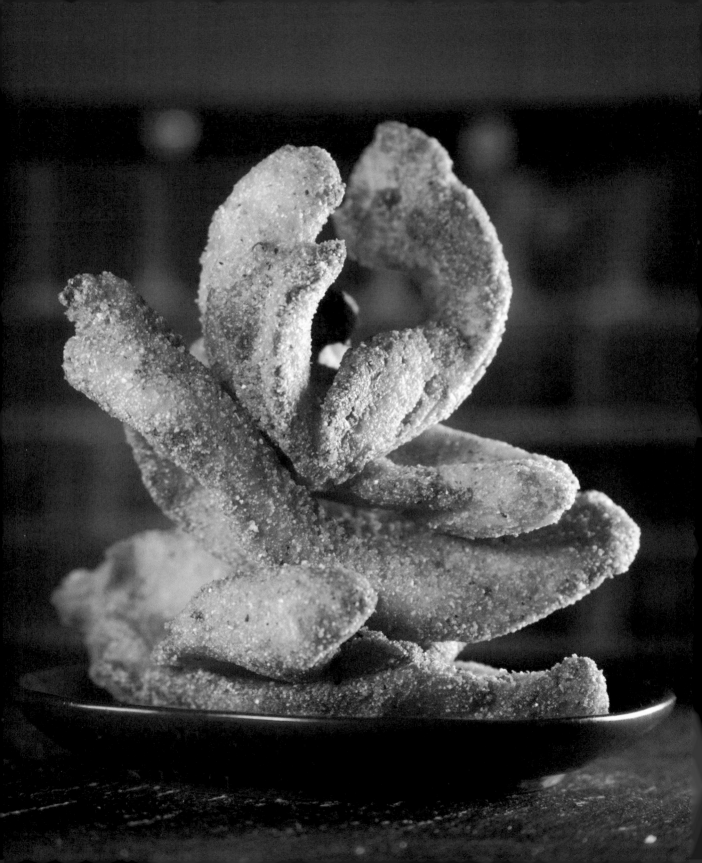

Pinewood Crispy Fish

Makes 4 servings

HERE IN THE SOUTH, you can find a fish fry just about anywhere, but finding one that's gluten free, well that's where Pinewood comes in. I was determined to create an old-school fish fry with all the traditional fixin's. Traditionally, a fish fry is made with catfish, but you can use any type of white fish you like.

4 large orange roughy filets, fresh *or* frozen and thawed*

1 onion, chopped medium

4 cloves garlic

¼ teaspoon sea salt *(or to taste)*

¼ teaspoon freshly ground black pepper *(or to taste)*

½ cup grapeseed oil *or* coconut oil

1 cup organic cornmeal, seasoned with sea salt and black pepper**

Substitutions:

*You can use any type of fish. A white fish is my favorite 'cause it turns out the best.

**If corn free, use almond meal.

1) Place the fish in a baking dish.

2) In a mini food processor, process the onion, garlic, sea salt, and black pepper until smooth. Pour over the fish to marinate. Cover the baking dish and place it in the refrigerator for several hours.

3) In a cast-iron skillet, heat up the oil. Dip the marinated fish in the seasoned cornmeal for a light dusting on both sides and drop it in the hot oil. Cook about 4 to 5 minutes per side. Watch closely because the fish cooks up pretty fast.

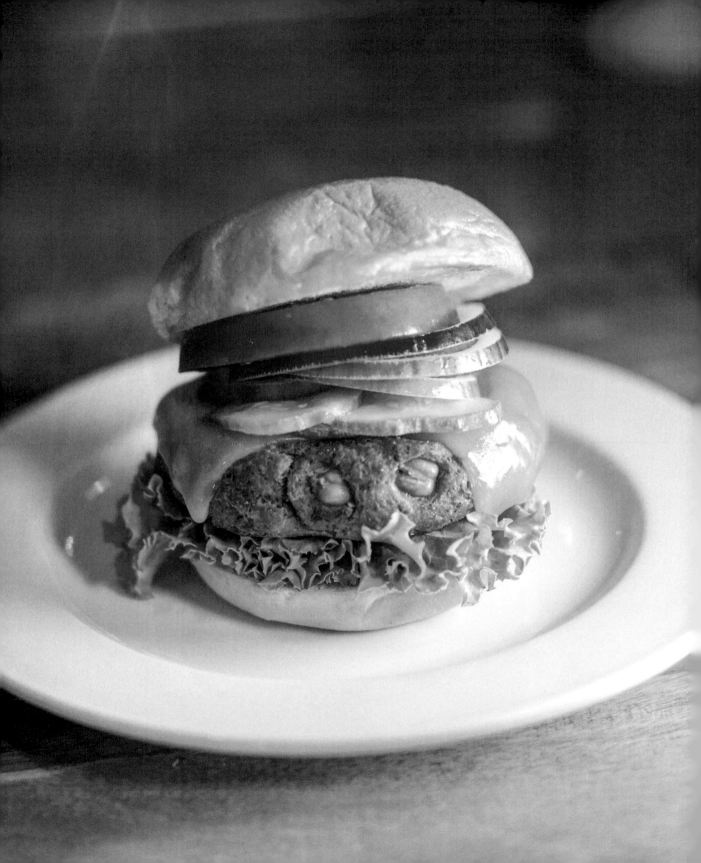

Full-On Falafel Burger

Makes 2 servings

BEFORE LIFE BROUGHT me to Pinewood, I spent a great deal of time in Israel. Falafel became one of my favorite comfort foods, so I brought it with me to Pinewood. It's one of our top sellers, and it warms my heart that so many have fallen in love with it. You can use this recipe to make classic falafel balls or you can make this full-on falafel burger that's such a big hit. Serve it on a gluten-free bun with your fixin's of choice.

Important Tip:
If you have weak digestion, soak the chickpeas overnight and cook them, removing the foam as they cook. If you use canned chickpeas, rinse them really well.

1 cup dried chickpeas, soaked overnight and drained *or* 1 cup canned chickpeas, rinsed well

½ large onion, roughly chopped

4 tablespoons finely chopped fresh parsley

1 teaspoon sea salt

½ to 1 teaspoon red pepper flakes *(optional)*

4 cloves garlic

1 teaspoon ground cumin

1 teaspoon baking powder

4 to 6 tablespoons chickpea flour *or* 1-to-1 gluten-free flour blend

About 8 cups grapeseed oil

1) In a food processor, combine the chickpeas, onion, parsley, sea salt, red pepper, garlic, and cumin. Process until blended but not pureed. (The mixture should not be smooth like hummus; it should have texture.)

2) Sprinkle in the baking powder and 4 tablespoons of the flour, and pulse. Add enough flour so that the dough is no longer sticky and can be formed into a burger or small balls. Place the chickpea mixture in a bowl, cover, and refrigerate for several hours.

3) Form the chickpea mixture into burger patties. In a deep pot, bring 3 inches of the grapeseed oil to 375°F. Cook for a few minutes on each side, or until golden brown. Drain on paper towels.

Sautéed Tofu

Makes 4 to 6 servings

THE LONGER YOU marinate the tofu, the better. Sometimes, I leave it in the fridge for 24 hours. The longer it marinates, the yummier it gets. This is great served over udon noodles with cabbage and carrots, or the next day in a gluten-free wrap.

1 *(14-ounce)* package organic tofu, washed

3 tablespoons tamari

2 tablespoons mirin *(rice wine)*

2 tablespoons grated fresh ginger

1 tablespoon sesame oil

1 tablespoon brown rice syrup

1 clove garlic

2 teaspoons sesame oil, organic peanut oil, *or* coconut oil

1) Steam the tofu for 15 minutes. Meanwhile, in a food processor, combine the remaining ingredients, except the sautéing oil.

2) Transfer the tofu to a dish and pour the marinade on top. Cover the dish and place it in the refrigerator. Let it marinate for several hours or up to 24 hours.

3) Heat a large skillet over medium-high heat. Add the oil, and when hot, sauté the tofu until it reaches the desired crispness.

Let's Tofu About It

Tofu is a soybean curd that originated in China thousands of years ago to improve the digestibility of the highly valued soybean. Some people think that the soy in tofu is bad for our health. The fact is, we do have way too much soy in our diets because it's become the fabric of processed foods. So if we eliminate processed foods and eat soy in its healthiest form—that is, non-GMO and pesticide free—including miso, tofu, tempeh, tamari/shoyu sauces (shoyu has gluten), and black soybeans, it can be good for us.

Tofu is full of B vitamins and minerals, including calcium, phosphorus, iron, sodium, and potassium. It's inexpensive, and if it is made right, the calcium levels can match those of dairy milk. Tofu has healing properties, too. It's known to relieve inflammation of the stomach and neutralize toxins. Cooking with it is a breeze since tofu is a flavor sponge. Always steam your tofu, even if you plan to sauté it. This makes it easier to digest and cuts down on the gas factor, especially if you have any digestive issues.

Coconut Bacon

Makes 2 cups

I LOVE BACON, BUT IT doesn't always love me back. The high fat can be tough for me to digest and I like to be mindful of how much animal I'm consuming. Coconut bacon is a great vegan/vegetarian and alpha-gal allergy friendly alternative added to veggies and salads. Top your dairy-free mac & cheez with this yumminess and you'll be in food nirvana.

2 cups large-flake unsweetened coconut

1 tablespoon avocado oil *or* grapeseed oil

2 tablespoons tamari *or* coconut aminos

1 teaspoon smoked paprika

1 tablespoon maple syrup

½ teaspoon organic liquid smoke

Pinch sea salt

½ teaspoon black pepper

1) Preheat the oven to 325°F.

2) Line a baking sheet with parchment paper. In a medium mixing bowl, combine the coconut flakes, oil, tamari or coconut aminos, paprika, maple syrup, liquid smoke, sea salt, and black pepper. Toss well so that all the coconut is coated.

3) Bake for 5 to 6 minutes, and then stir and flip the pan around. Bake for another 5 to 6 minutes until the coconut bacon is crispy and golden brown. Watch carefully so that it doesn't burn.

4) Remove from the oven and allow it to rest. Store it in a glass jar.

Tempeh Bacon

Makes about 24 strips

TEMPEH IS ONE OF MY favorite meat alternatives and it's excellent served in a sandwich as a T.L.T.

2 *(8-ounce)* packages gluten-free organic tempeh*

½ cup tamari or coconut aminos

½ cup apple cider vinegar

2 tablespoons pure maple syrup *or* local honey**

½ teaspoon ground cumin

2 teaspoons organic liquid smoke

Substitutions:

*If soy free, use hemp tempeh.

**If watching sugar, replace with an equivalent amount of stevia *(page 51)*.

1) Slice the tempeh into ¼-inch slices. You will get about 12 strips per package of tempeh, or 24 total.

2) In a medium bowl, whisk together the tamari or coconut aminos, apple cider vinegar, maple syrup or honey, ground cumin, and liquid smoke.

3) Place the tempeh strips in a dish, and cover with the marinade. Make sure the strips are well coated. Cover and marinate in the refrigerator for at least an hour.

4) Preheat the oven to 350°F.

5) Line a large baking sheet with parchment paper. Place the marinated tempeh strips on the baking sheet. Bake for 15 minutes. Flip each piece and bake for 15 more minutes.

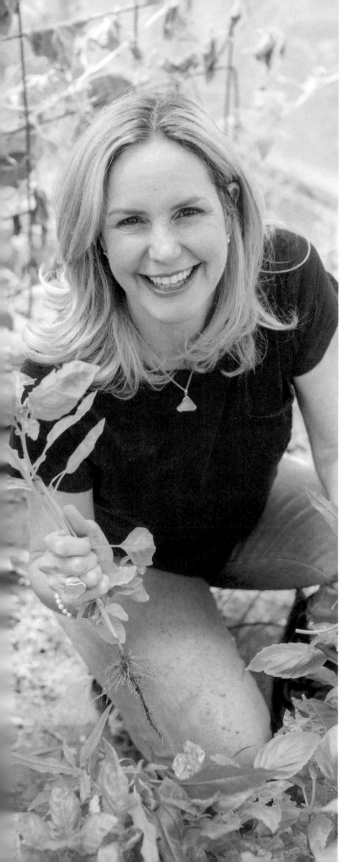

Veggies To Make Your Gut Happy

We should all try to eat a rainbow of vegetables each and every week. Often, though, we get busy, and some folks tell me they get stuck in a cooking rut, making the same sides every week. It's my hope that these recipes encourage you to try some new vegetables and some new ways to prepare them. If you start your kids early eating their greens (and purples, and whites, and yellows), they will grow to love their vegetables.

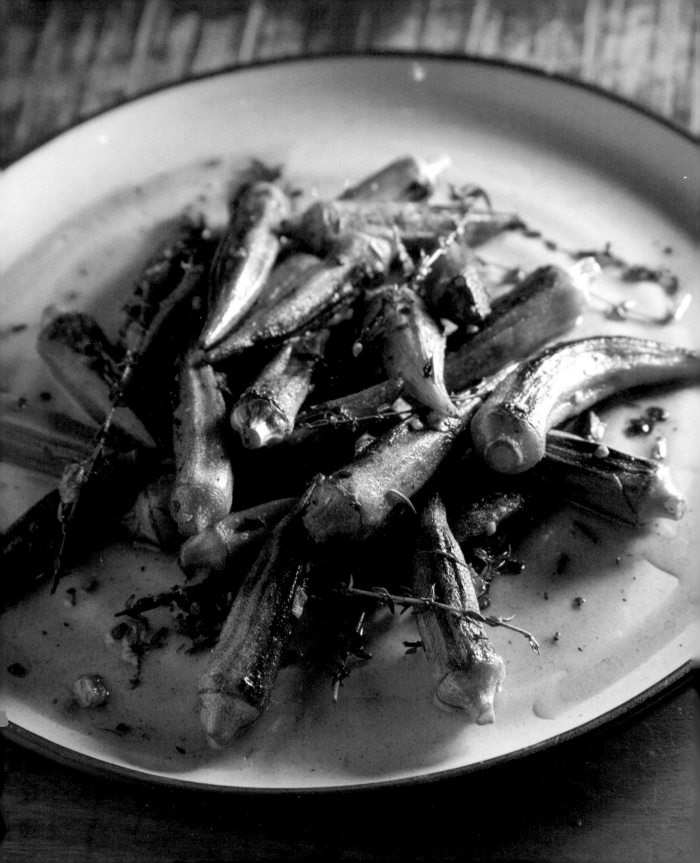

Roasted Okra

Makes 4 servings

WE GROW OKRA ON THE FARM and when it arrives we go okra crazy. We pickle it, fry it, stew it, and roast it. Roasting is the easiest way to cook it, and it removes the "sliminess" associated with okra. I can eat my weight in roasted okra—it's that good.

18 fresh okra pods, sliced in rounds *or* whole

2 tablespoons extra-virgin olive oil

2 teaspoons sea salt

Freshly ground black pepper *(to taste)*

1) Preheat the oven to 425°F. Line a baking sheet with parchment paper.

2) In a large bowl, combine the okra, oil, and sea salt. Toss to coat well.

3) Transfer the okra to the baking sheet, and roast for 12 to 15 minutes, until crispy, but not charred. Season with black pepper, to taste.

Trimmin' Kale

To trim the kale, grab each stem with one hand and rip the two leafy sides away from it with the other hand. Or fold the leaf in half and a run a knife down the inside seam, cutting away the stem. Discard the stems, as they can be hard to digest. I like to cut kale into bite-size pieces, but you can leave them whole if it suits your use.

Tuscan Kale with Shallots and Crisp Organic Salami

Makes 4 servings

2 ounces nitrate-free organic Genoa salami*

2 teaspoons local honey, coconut sugar, *or* monk sugar**

1 teaspoon sherry vinegar

1 tablespoon sea salt, plus more, to taste

14 ounces Tuscan kale *(aka Lacinato kale)*, trimmed and torn into bite-size pieces

2 teaspoons extra-virgin olive oil

2 large or 4 small shallots *(about 4 ounces)*, sliced into thin rings

Substitutions:

*If meat free, replace with 2 medium carrots, cut into ribbons, and sautéed in oil till crispy, about 5 minutes.

**If watching sugar, replace with an equivalent amount of stevia *(page 51)*.

1) Cut the salami into ⅛- to ¼-inch wide strips.

2) In a small bowl, whisk together the honey, coconut sugar, or monk sugar and vinegar. Set aside.

3) Fill a 5- to 6-quart pot about three-quarters full with water. Add the sea salt and bring to a boil over high heat. Add the kale to the boiling water and cook until just tender, about 4 to 7 minutes. Drain and spread the kale out on a rimmed baking sheet to dry.

4) In a large nonstick skillet, heat the olive oil over medium heat. Add the shallot rings and cook, stirring with a wooden spoon, until soft and lightly browned, about 4 minutes. Transfer the shallots to a plate.

5) Increase the heat to medium-high, add the salami strips, and cook, stirring and breaking them up into smaller bits, until crisp, about 2 minutes. Transfer the salami to a plate.

6) Add the kale to the pan and toss with the olive oil just until the kale is heated through. (Do not cook it for long or it will begin to weep moisture.) Take the kale off the heat, transfer to a serving bowl, and add the honey mixture. Toss well. Season with sea salt to taste. Garnish with the salami or carrot ribbons.

SUMMERTIME MEANS OODLES OF ZOODLES.
I use zucchini or squash—whatever the garden
gives us. I love topping my pasta with grilled or
sautéed mushrooms. This pasta recipe travels well, so
it's perfect for summer potlucks or picnics.
The addition of vitamin B–rich nutritional
yeast along with probiotic miso
gives the pesto a cheezy
taste without the dairy.

Zucchini Spaghetti Noodles with Dairy-Free Pesto

Makes 4 servings

4 small zucchini, ends trimmed*

1 cup packed fresh basil leaves

2 cloves garlic, peeled

2 teaspoons fresh lemon juice

1 tablespoon nutritional yeast

½ teaspoon miso

1 cup pine nuts**

Sea salt *(to taste)*

Freshly ground black pepper *(to taste)*

⅓ cup extra-virgin olive oil

½ cup sliced cherry *or* grape tomatoes *(optional)*

Substitutions:

*If short on time, buy pre-cut zucchini noodles in your market.

**If nut free, replace with pumpkin seeds.

1) Using a veggie spiralizer, a julienne peeler, or a mandoline slicer, slice the zucchini into noodles. Set aside.

2) In a blender or food processor, combine the basil, garlic, lemon juice, nutritional yeast, miso, pine nuts, sea salt, and black pepper, and pulse until coarsely chopped.

3) Slowly add the olive oil in a constant stream while the blender or food processor is running. Stop the machine and scrape down the sides with a rubber spatula. Pulse until blended.

4) Transfer the zucchini noodles to a serving bowl and add the pesto. Toss until the zucchini noodles are well coated. Top with the tomatoes (if using). Serve at room temperature or chilled. Alternatively, transfer the zucchini pesto noodles to a skillet and sauté them over medium heat for 4 to 5 minutes, and serve hot.

NO DOUBT THIS IS THE BEST VEGGIE-BASED
mac and cheez I've had. It's so satisfying and fulfills
my cravings for my old food favorites with new
healthier alternatives. This recipe is loaded with
good gut-supporting ingredients.

Super Creamy Veggie Mac and Cheez

Makes 5 to 6 servings

16 ounces gluten-free penne pasta *or* any type of gluten-free pasta

1 tablespoon vegan butter

⅓ cup diced onions

2 cups diced carrots

1½ cups peeled and diced yellow potatoes*

1 teaspoon crushed garlic

½ cup raw cashews

¼ cup whole-fat coconut milk, unsweetened oat milk, *or* unsweetened hemp milk

¼ cup nutritional yeast

½ teaspoon sea salt

1 tablespoon fresh lemon juice

2 tablespoons miso

Pinch cayenne

Pinch paprika

1 tablespoon chopped fresh chives for garnish *(optional)*

Substitutions:

*If avoiding potatoes, replace with 1½ cups of cooked quinoa.

1) Cook the pasta according to the package instructions, being careful not to overcook. Remove the pasta from the water and place in a serving bowl. Reserve 3 cups of the starchy cooking water.

2) In a heated saucepan, melt the butter and sauté the onions until soft; add the carrots, potatoes, and garlic. Add 2 cups of leftover cooking water. Add the raw cashews, milk, and nutritional yeast, sea salt, and lemon juice. Simmer until the veggies are soft, about 15 minutes.

3) Transfer the vegetables to a blender or food processor. Add the miso and blend until completely smooth. If the sauce seems too thick, add the reserved cooking water a little at a time to reach the desired consistency.

4) Pour the sauce over the pasta and season with the cayenne and paprika. Sprinkle with the chives (if using).

Variation: *If you want to take your mac and cheez to the next level, transfer it to a baking dish, top with a handful of gluten-free panko crumbs or almond meal, and bake at 350°F for 15 minutes until the topping is golden brown. Then season with paprika and cayenne, and sprinkle on the chives.*

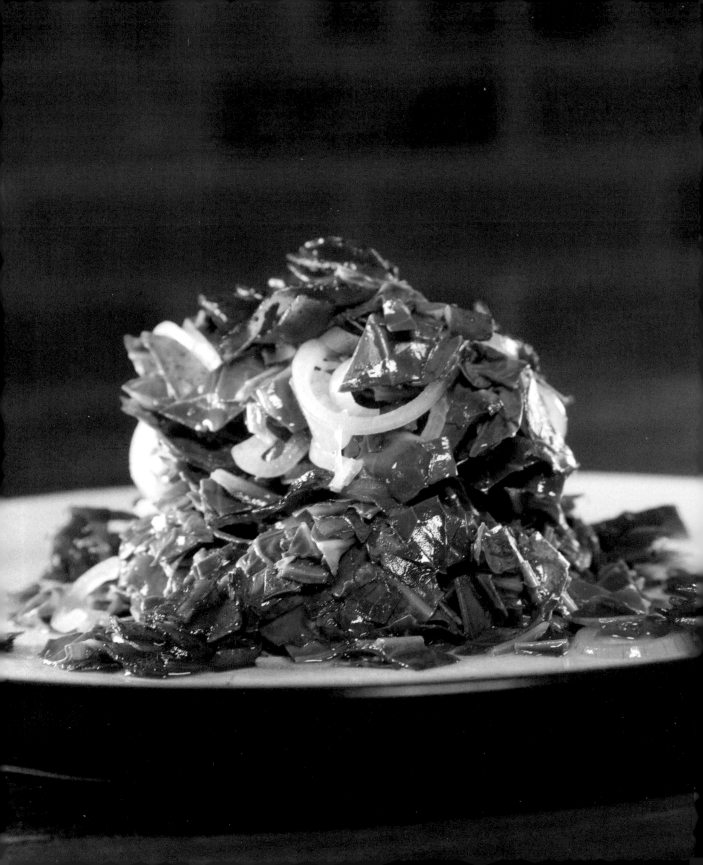

Speedy Collards with Coconut Bacon and Onions

Makes 4 servings

I'D ALWAYS THOUGHT of collards as being soggy overcooked greens, but this recipe is bright and fresh. My husband loves it with crispy pork bacon, but I prefer adding coconut bacon to give it an inclusive yet Southern twist.

1 to 2 tablespoons extra-virgin olive oil

1 small yellow onion, chopped

2 pounds collards, stemmed and sliced into ¾-inch ribbons

¼ cup white vinegar

½ cup water

⅓ cup Coconut Bacon *(page 157)**

Sea salt *(to taste)*

Freshly ground black pepper *(to taste)*

Substitutions:

*If you like pork *or* turkey bacon, feel free to use it instead.

1) In a large Dutch oven over medium heat, heat up the oil and sauté the onion, until soft and brown in spots, about 5 minutes.

2) Add the collards, vinegar, and water to the pot. Cook, stirring occasionally, until wilted and tender, about 20 minutes. Add the coconut bacon and stir. Season with sea salt and black pepper, to taste.

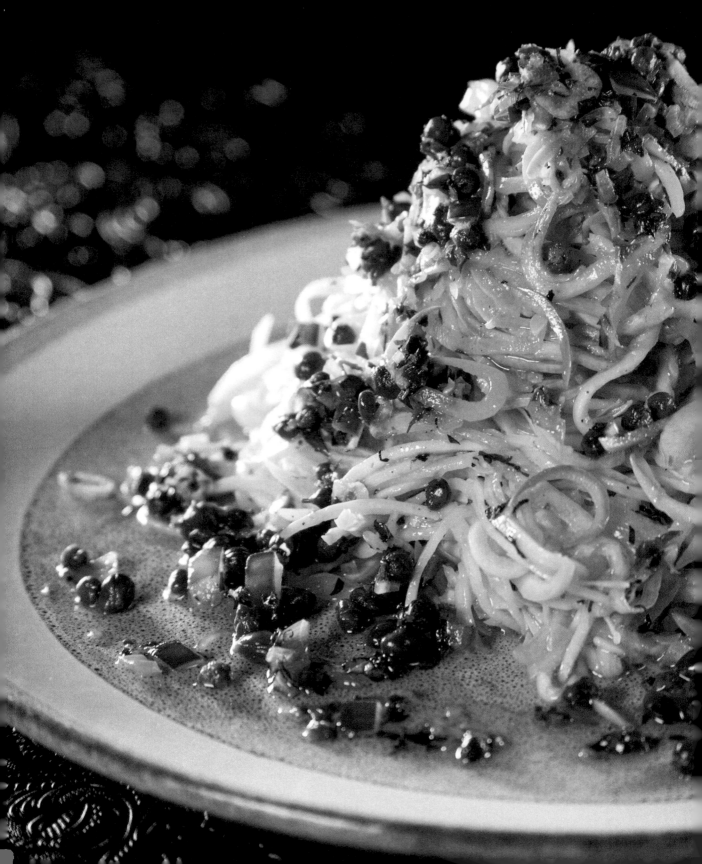

Zephyr Squash Ribbons with Almond Salsa Verde

Makes 6 servings

THE BEAUTY OF A SUMMER garden is that every week we welcome an old friend we've not seen since the previous summer to the table. Zephyr squash is beautiful because it looks as if someone tie-dyed the bottom green and the top yellow. It's mild and delicious. You can use any summer squash or zucchini in this recipe. Summer squashes have a lot of water in them, which aids digestion. I also rotate the nuts that I use in this recipe.

½ cup finely chopped toasted blanched almonds*

¼ cup finely chopped fresh cilantro

¼ cup finely chopped fresh flat-leaf parsley

¼ cup extra-virgin olive oil plus more for drizzling

2 tablespoons fresh lemon juice

1½ tablespoons chopped capers

1 tablespoon minced shallots

1 teaspoon minced garlic

¼ teaspoon sea salt, plus more *(to taste)*

1¼ pounds summer squash *or* green zucchini, trimmed and cut in half crosswise

Freshly ground black pepper *(to taste)*

Substitutions:

*If nut free, replace with pumpkin seeds.

1) To make the salsa verde: In a large bowl, combine the almonds, cilantro, parsley, olive oil, lemon juice, capers, shallots, garlic, and sea salt. Toss until well combined.

2) Shave the squash into ribbons using a vegetable peeler. Transfer to a serving bowl and toss with the salsa verde. Season with sea salt and black pepper, to taste. Drizzle with some extra-virgin olive oil.

Sweet Potato and Apple Casserole with a Pecan Crust

Makes 8 servings

THIS IS ONE OF MY all-time favorite recipes. Granny Smith apples are a super prebiotic food, sweet potatoes are loaded with vitamin C, and pecans make me so happy — plus they, too, are considered a super nut for the gut.

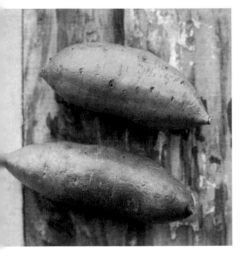

FOR THE PECAN CRUST:

1 cup toasted and very finely chopped pecans

2 tablespoons grass-fed butter *or* ghee*

3 tablespoons coconut sugar

1⅓ cups almond flour**

Substitutions:

*If dairy free, replace with vegan butter.

**If nut free, replace with gluten-free breadcrumbs.

FOR THE CASSEROLE:

3 large sweet potatoes

4 tablespoons grass-fed butter *or* ghee, plus more for the pan*

1 cup full-fat coconut cream *or* any nondairy cream

2 tablespoons local honey**

8 ¼-inch thick slices fresh ginger, unpeeled and crushed

2 whole star anise

1 *(2- to 3-inch)* cinnamon stick

2 tablespoons plus 2 teaspoons rum***

1½ teaspoons pure vanilla extract

½ teaspoon sea salt, divided

3 large Granny Smith apples, peeled, quartered, cored, and thinly sliced

1) In a food processor, combine the pecans, butter or ghee, sugar, and almond flour, and pulse three or four times. Transfer the mixture into a bowl and blend with your hands. Set aside.

2) Position a rack in the center of the oven and preheat the oven to 400°F. Line a rimmed baking sheet with aluminum foil.

3) Prick the sweet potatoes all over with a fork and bake them on the sheet until completely tender when pierced with a fork, about 55 to 60 minutes. Let them rest until cool enough to handle. Reduce the oven temperature to 375°F.

4) Discard the potato skins and transfer the flesh to a medium mixing bowl. Add 2 tablespoons of the butter. With a potato masher, work the sweet potatoes until they're well mashed (they don't have to be perfectly smooth).

5) Combine the cream, honey, ginger, star anise, and cinnamon stick in a small saucepan. Bring to a full boil (watch carefully so that it doesn't boil over) and remove from the heat immediately. Let it steep for 15 to 20 minutes. Strain through a fine sieve into a liquid measuring cup, pressing down on the solids with a spatula to extract all the liquid. Stir in 2 tablespoons of the bourbon or rum, vanilla extract, and ¼ teaspoon of the sea salt.

6) In a 12-inch nonstick skillet over medium-high heat, melt the remaining 2 tablespoons butter. Add the apples, season with the remaining sea salt, and toss well. Raise the heat to high and cook, stirring frequently, until the apples are soft and lightly browned, about 8 to 9 minutes. Lower the heat if the apples are getting too dark, but not so much that they soften without browning.

7) Turn off the heat. Carefully add the 2 teaspoons of the bourbon or rum, and stir for a few seconds until it evaporates. Pour in ⅓ cup of the infused cream and stir until the apples have absorbed most of it, a few more seconds. Set the pan aside and let the apples cool for about 15 minutes, turning them occasionally to release steam.

8) To assemble the casserole, butter a 12-inch cast-iron skillet or a shallow 3-quart baking dish. Add the remaining cream to the mashed sweet potatoes and mix thoroughly. Season with additional sea salt to taste, if desired. Arrange the apples across the bottom of the baking dish. Spread the sweet potato mixture over the apples in an even layer. Top with the pecan-crumb mixture.

9) Bake the casserole at 375°F until the crumb topping is dark brown (it will be browner around the edges) and the casserole is heated through, about 25 minutes.

BLACK-EYED PEAS ARE CONSIDERED GOOD LUCK IF EATEN ON NEW YEAR'S DAY,
so I serve this dish every New Year's in the restaurant as an appetizer and in my farmhouse to friends and family as hors d'oeuvres. If you have weak digestion, be sure to use fully cooked black-eyed peas as this recipe calls for soaked-only peas. I serve them with a dollop of probiotic miso-turmeric sauce and fresh parsley.

Black-Eyed Pea Croquettes

Makes 12 small croquettes

FOR THE CROQUETTES:

2 cups dried black-eyed peas

1 piece kombu

½ teaspoon sea salt

1 teaspoon tamari *or* coconut aminos

1 teaspoon ground cumin

2 cups coconut oil

FOR THE DIPPING SAUCE:

1 heaping tablespoon miso

¼ onion, chopped small

1 clove fresh garlic

½ cup grapeseed oil, Basic Mayo *(page 212)*, *or* Vegan Mayo *(page 213)*

3 tablespoons water

Freshly ground black pepper *(to taste)*

FOR THE DRIZZLE:

½ cup brown rice syrup

1 to 2 tablespoons Dijon mustard

⅛ cup chopped parsley *or* cilantro *(for garnish)*

1) Soak the black-eyed peas in spring water with a piece of kombu overnight. Drain and rinse.

2) To make the dipping sauce, combine all the ingredients in a food processor or blender, and blend until smooth and creamy. Pour into a dish and set aside until ready to serve.

3) Place the black-eyed peas in the food processor. Add the sea salt, tamari, and cumin. Blend until there are fine shreds of bean (don't blend into a pulp). The mixture will be slightly wet but it will still hold together. Using your hands, form palm-size croquettes.

4) Heat 1 inch of oil in a cast-iron skillet to about 350°F. To test the oil, drop in a tiny amount of the croquette mixture. If it bubbles furiously and rises to the top, the oil is ready. Do not let the oil get so hot that it smokes. You may need to make small adjustments to the heat throughout the cooking process to avoid burning the croquettes.

5) Place four croquettes in the oil and let them fry for about 4 minutes on each side. Transfer the cooked croquettes to a paper towel to drain excess oil.

6) In a small pot, heat the brown rice syrup and mustard over low heat until it bubbles. Drizzle onto the serving dish. Arrange the croquettes on top of the syrup and garnish with the parsley or cilantro. Serve alongside the dipping sauce.

Kinpira Gobo

Makes 4 to 6 servings

KINPIRA GOBO IS A GET-DOWN good veggie dish that combines burdock root and carrots. Burdock root is known to fight inflammation and strengthen the blood, and it's excellent for teens with acne.

Splash of brown rice vinegar *(optional)*

2 burdock roots, scrubbed well and julienned *or* sliced into discs

2 tablespoons sesame oil

2 small or 1 medium carrot, peeled and julienned *or* sliced into discs

1 teaspoon red chili pepper flakes *or* 2 small fresh red chili peppers, finely chopped *(optional)*

2 tablespoons mirin *(rice wine)*

2 to 3 tablespoons tamari *or* coconut aminos

½ cup water

1) As an optional first step, place the burdock root pieces in a bowl with enough water and a splash of brown rice vinegar to cover. Let them soak for a few minutes. Drain away the water, and refill the bowl with fresh water. Soak for a few minutes more and then drain again. Soaking burdock isn't necessary, but it will prevent discoloration and will give a milder flavor. Pat the burdock root dry.

2) Heat up a wok or large frying pan over high heat with the sesame oil. Add the burdock root and carrot pieces and sauté briefly. Add the chili pepper (if using) and toss. Add the mirin and tamari or coconut aminos and the water. Lower the heat to medium, and continue stirring until the moisture has disappeared.

3) Taste a piece for doneness: it should be crisp-tender. If it's too crunchy for you, add a bit more water and cook a bit longer.

Turn Up the Greens

Makes 4 servings

TURNIPS MAKE ME HAPPY AND OUR GUT BACTERIA SUPA-DUPA HAPPY. ADDITIONALLY,
turnips regulate metabolism, lower inflammation, increase circulation, and boost the immune system.
Most folks just eat the greens, but by eating all the parts, including the turnip, we benefit from all the
goodness of the plant in one dish. A little sweetener cuts the bitter taste, but it's not necessary.

1 medium onion, chopped

2 tablespoons extra-virgin olive oil

2¾ pounds peeled turnips, cut into ½-inch cubes

12 ounces fresh turnip greens

3 cups broth of choice

4 tablespoons apple cider vinegar

1¼ teaspoons sea salt

1½ teaspoons coarsely ground black pepper

3 tablespoons local honey *(optional)**

2 smoked ham hocks *(optional)***

Substitutions:

*If watching sugar, replace with an equivalent amount of stevia *(page 51)*.

**If meat free, omit the ham hocks and sprinkle with Coconut Bacon before serving *(page 157)*.

STOVETOP DIRECTIONS:

1) In a large pot over medium heat, sauté the onion in the olive oil until soft.

2) Add the turnips, turnip greens, broth, vinegar, sea salt, and black pepper.

3) Add the honey (if using) and the ham hocks (if using). Cook for about 20 minutes.

4) Remove the ham hock from the dish. Remove the meat from the bones when cool enough to handle; cut the ham into small pieces and return to the pot. Serve warm with a slotted spoon.

PRESSURE COOKER DIRECTIONS:

1) In a 6-quart electric pressure cooker, combine all the ingredients. Lock the lid; make sure the vent is closed. Select the "manual" setting; adjust the pressure to high and set the time for 5 minutes.

2) When finished cooking, allow the pressure to naturally release for 10 minutes, then quick-release the remaining pressure according to the manufacturer's directions.

3) If using ham hocks, remove the meat from the bones when cool enough to handle; cut the ham into small pieces and return to the pressure cooker. Serve warm with a slotted spoon.

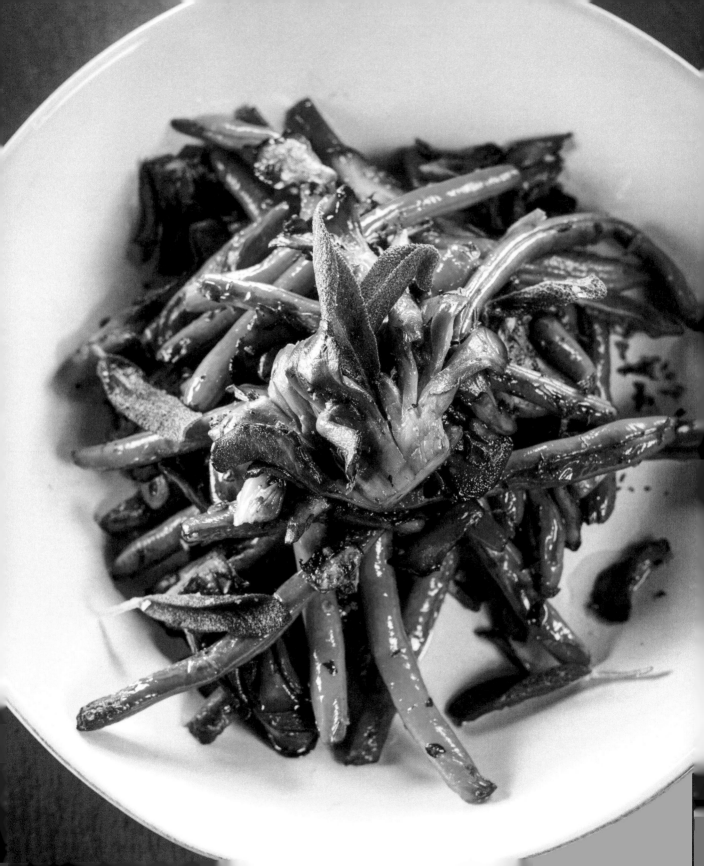

Sage & Maitake Green Beans

Makes 4 servings

THIS RECIPE CAN BE made with any mushroom, but my goal is to inspire you to try them all. I love maitake mushrooms; they have a mild, woodsy flavor that melds well with earthy fresh sage. Sage is one of the most powerful healing herbs, and the combination of all these ingredients supports gut, immune, and vascular health.

1 pound organic green beans, trimmed and cut into 2-inch pieces

2 tablespoons vegan butter, grass-fed butter, *or* ghee*

2 tablespoons extra-virgin olive oil

½ cup fresh sage leaves

1 maitake mushroom, chopped

3 garlic cloves, minced

½ cup Chicken Bone Broth *(page 120) or* Vegetable Broth *(page 121)*

2 tablespoons white wine *(optional)*

1 tablespoon tamari *or* coconut aminos

½ teaspoon sea salt

¼ teaspoon black pepper

1) Cook the beans in boiling sea-salted water for 8 minutes or until crisp-tender; drain. Plunge into ice water to stop the cooking process; drain and set aside.

2) In a large skillet over medium-high heat, melt the butter with the olive oil. Add the sage and sauté for 1 minute or until crisp and dark green. Remove with a slotted spoon and set aside.

3) In the same skillet, add the maitake mushrooms and garlic; sauté for about 3 minutes until the liquid evaporates. Add the green beans, tossing to combine. Stir in the broth and the remaining ingredients. Stir in the sage just before serving.

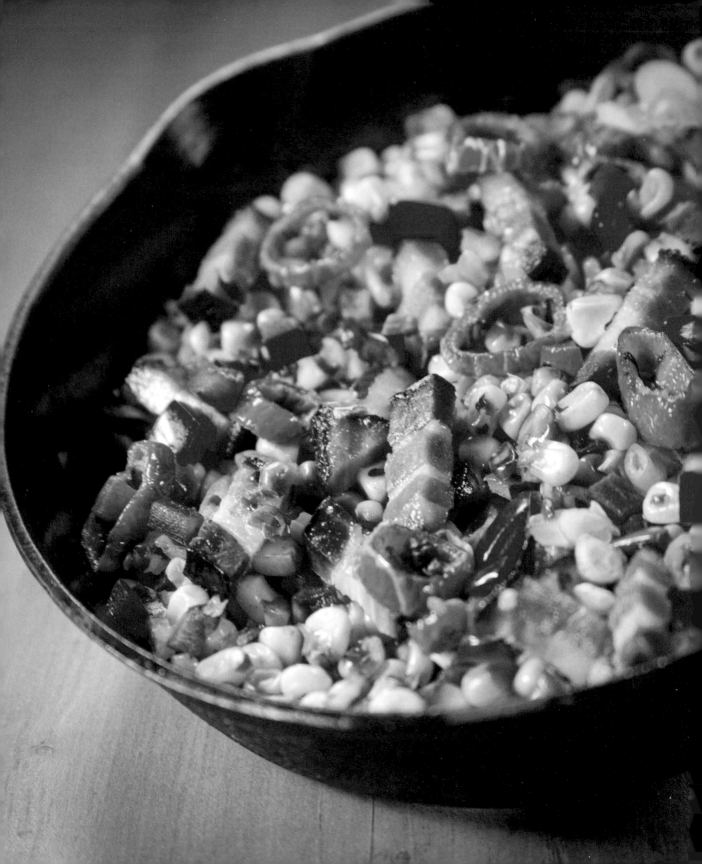

Fried Corn with Bacon & Fresh Jalapeños

Makes 4 to 6 servings

FRIED CORN IS

crazy good. I grew up eating creamed corn out of a can. When our corn started growing, I started dreaming of how to make a better version of creamed corn without the heavy cream, and this is my alternative. I know corn isn't for everyone, but if you are able to eat it, give this a try. It's great served with chopped avocado or avocado slices.

4 strips bacon*

1 tablespoon extra-virgin olive oil *or* coconut oil

1 cup diced red onion

3 cloves crushed garlic

1 cup diced red bell pepper

2 fresh jalapeños seeded, deveined, and diced

3 cups fresh corn kernels sliced off the cob *(about 6 to 8 ears)*

2 tablespoons local honey *or* 2 tablespoons maple syrup**

3 tablespoons apple cider vinegar

Dash sea salt

Red pepper flakes *(to taste)*

Substitutions:

*If meat free, replace with Coconut Bacon *(page 157)* or Tempeh Bacon *(page 158)*.

**If watching sugar, replace with an equivalent amount of stevia *(page 51)*.

1) In a medium skillet, fry the bacon in the oil until crispy; transfer to a paper towel to drain.

2) Add the onion, garlic, red pepper, and jalapeños to the skillet and cook until soft, about 4 minutes.

3) Add the corn and cook until soft. Crumble the bacon and toss in with the corn.

4) Remove from the heat and stir in the honey and apple cider vinegar. Season with sea salt and some red pepper flakes, to taste, for extra heat.

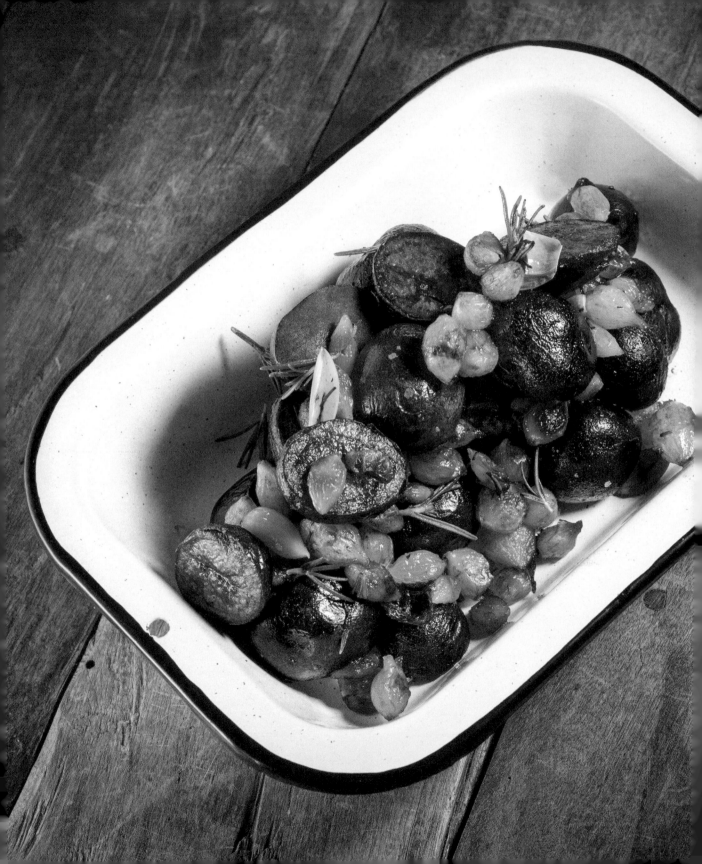

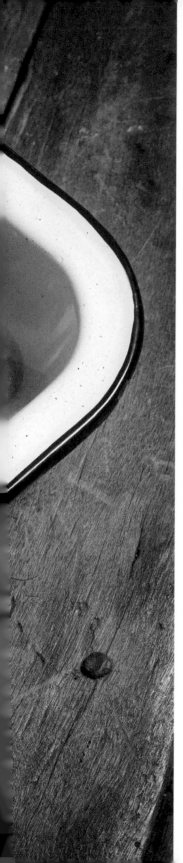

Roasted Purple Potatoes and Pearl Onions

Makes 4 servings

GETTING MY KIDS to eat something other than white mashed potatoes started right here with this recipe, as it's a fantastic way to introduce color and herbs.

Grapeseed oil cooking spray

3 pounds purple *or* red potatoes, scrubbed and cut into ½-inch pieces

1 *(10-ounce)* package pearl onions, peeled, *or* fresh pearled onions

2 tablespoons extra-virgin olive oil

2 teaspoons dried basil

1 teaspoon smoked paprika

¾ teaspoon sea salt

1 teaspoon finely chopped fresh rosemary

¾ teaspoon black pepper

1) Preheat the oven to 400°F. Spray a large, shallow roasting pan with nonstick grapeseed oil or coconut oil cooking spray.

2) Combine the potatoes and onions in the prepared pan. Drizzle with oil; toss to coat. Combine the basil, paprika, sea salt, rosemary, and black pepper in a small bowl; mix well. Sprinkle the mixture over the potatoes and onions; toss to coat.

3) Roast the potatoes and onions for 20 minutes. Stir and then roast for 15 to 20 minutes more or until the potatoes are browned and tender when pierced with a fork.

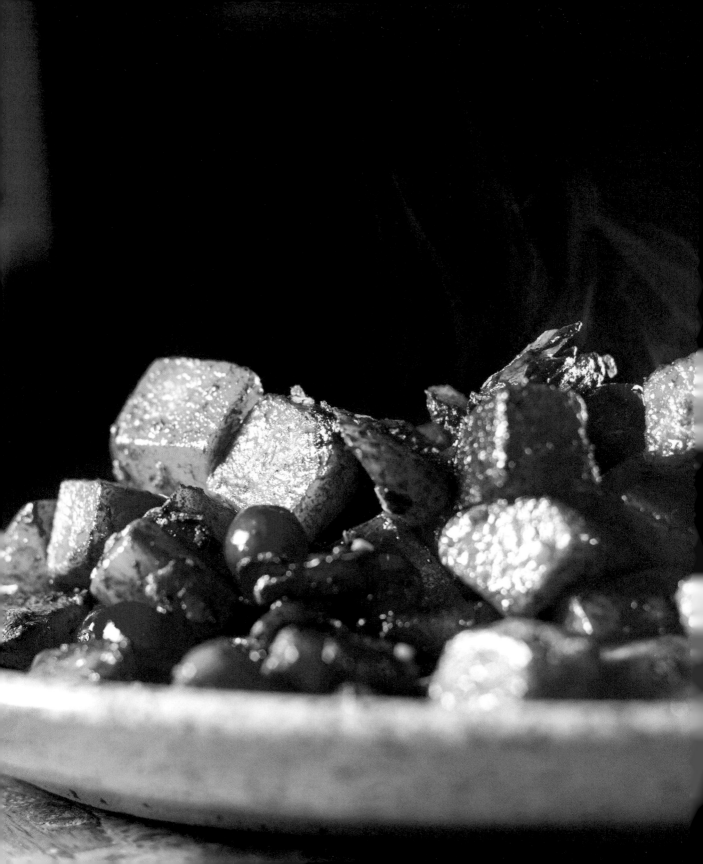

Balsamic Butternut Squash with Cranberries

Makes **4** servings

WHEN I WAS A KID, I could not stand butternut squash, but now it's one of my favorite foods. When I'm feeling out of sorts with the change of season or my digestion is on the struggle bus — which usually happens when I'm not grounded in my space and eating out more than I should — it's butternut squash to the rescue. This is also a perfect Thanksgiving dinner side dish.

3 tablespoons extra-virgin olive oil

2 tablespoons thinly sliced fresh sage *(about 6 large leaves)*, divided

½ red onion, halved and cut into ¼-inch slices

1 medium butternut squash, peeled and cut into 1-inch pieces

1 teaspoon sea salt, divided

¼ cup water *or* broth of choice

¼ cup dried cranberries, no sugar added

2½ tablespoons balsamic vinegar

¼ teaspoon black pepper

1) Heat the oil in a large cast-iron skillet over medium-high heat. Add 1 tablespoon of the sage; cook and stir for 3 minutes.

2) Add the onion and sauté it until is soft. Add the butternut squash, ½ teaspoon of the sea salt, and the water or broth. Cover with a lid and steam for 6 minutes, stirring occasionally. Reduce the heat to medium; cook for 10 minutes without stirring. Add the dried cranberries and cook for 5 minutes.

3) Add the vinegar, the remaining ½ teaspoon sea salt, and black pepper; cook for 10 minutes more or until the squash is tender, stirring occasionally. Stir in the remaining 1 tablespoon of sage; cook 1 minute more.

Pickled Okra

PICKLED OKRA GOES WELL on everything. We add it to our grain bowls, and serve it alongside burgers and fries and our fish baskets.

1½ pounds fresh okra

2 cups water

1 cup apple cider vinegar

¼ cup coconut sugar

2 tablespoons sea salt

1) Divide the okra evenly between three sterile 1-pint jars.

2) In a small saucepan, combine the water, vinegar, sugar, and sea salt. Bring to a boil, stirring constantly.

3) Lower the heat, and when the sugar and salt have dissolved, pour the mixture over the okra in the jars. Seal the lids and refrigerate.

Tip: *You can add a dash of red pepper flakes or a few slices of fresh chilis for a spicy pickled okra.*

Arame with Carrots

Makes 4 servings

WOULD YOU EVER THINK

to combine seaweed and carrots? The combination is surprisingly tasty, and this is a great way to introduce arame or any sea veggie to your family. Be sure not to use too much arame, or it will be like eating a bowl of beach!

½ cup arame *or* hijiki seaweed

1 tablespoon toasted sesame oil

1 small onion, thinly sliced

4 large carrots, peeled and julienned

2 tablespoons tamari *or* coconut aminos, divided

1 tablespoon mirin *(rice wine)*

2 scallions, thinly sliced

1 tablespoon toasted sesame seeds *(optional)*

1) Rinse the arame or hijiki in a mesh strainer, removing any debris and dirt, and then hydrate in a bowl of water for 10 minutes. Drain well.

2) In a large, heavy skillet over medium heat, heat the sesame oil. Add the onion and sauté for 5 minutes or until the onion is tender and beginning to brown. Add the drained arame or hijiki, the carrots, 1 tablespoon of the tamari or coconut aminos, and the mirin.

3) Decrease the heat to medium-low and sauté the mixture for 8 minutes. Stir in the remaining tablespoon of tamari or coconut aminos.

4) Transfer to a bowl and sprinkle with the scallions and sesame seeds (if using). Serve warm or cold.

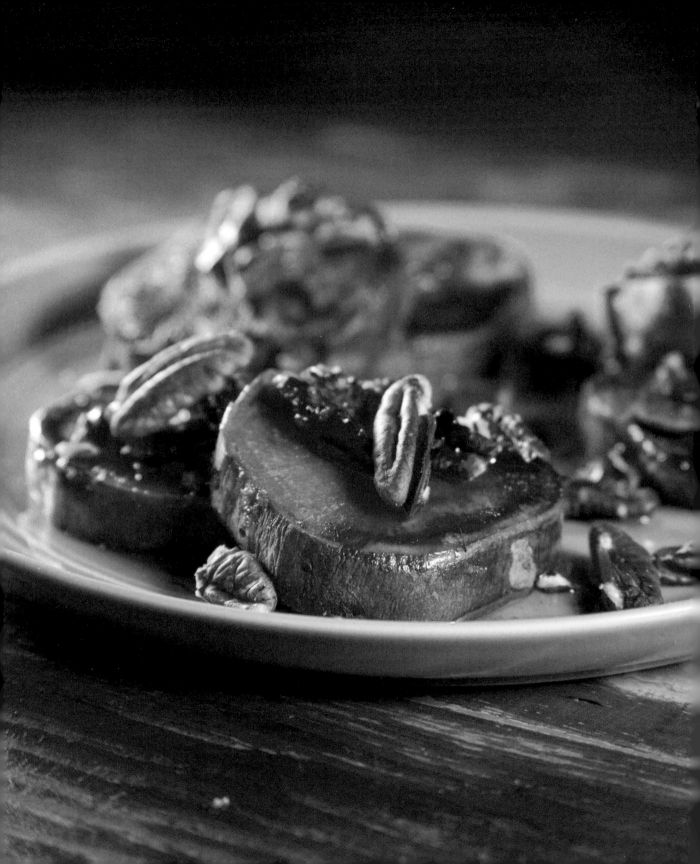

Coconut & Local Honey Sweet Potatoes

Makes 4 to 6 servings

THIS IS A GO-TO IN OUR house for dinner, but it also makes a great dessert. I like to add toasted pecans to really liven it up. I always recommend using a local honey because it actually helps fight against seasonal allergies. Skip it if you're avoiding honey, but if not, try to buy local. Depending on where our hives are located on the farm, the taste of the honey changes. We have a few hives next to the blueberries, and this gives them a hint of blueberry — my favorite!

¼ cup melted organic coconut oil, plus more for drizzling

2 tablespoons sesame oil

¼ cup local honey*

1 tablespoon tamari *or* coconut aminos

2 teaspoons ground cinnamon

4 sweet potatoes, cut into 1½-inch rounds

Dash coarse sea salt

¼ cup toasted, chopped pecans

Substitutions:

*If watching sugar, omit the honey.

1) Preheat the oven to 400°F.

2) In a large mixing bowl, combine the coconut oil, sesame oil, honey, tamari or coconut aminos, and cinnamon; add the sweet potatoes. Toss until well coated.

3) Arrange the sweet potatoes in a single layer on a roasting tray. Sprinkle with sea salt. Roast for 25 to 30 minutes or until tender.

4) Transfer the sweet potatoes to a serving platter. Drizzle with additional honey and coconut oil, if desired. Sprinkle with the pecans.

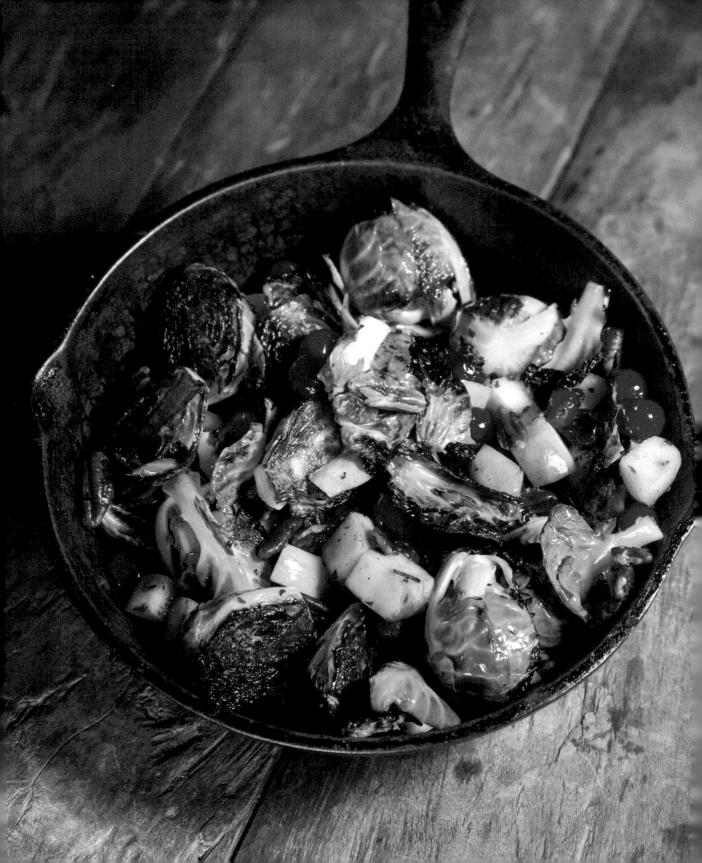

Celebration Brussels Sprouts

Makes 4 servings

BRUSSELS SPROUTS

are my jam, and we make them weekly in Pinewood when they are coming off the farm. I like them roasted with garlic and olive oil, but I know that folks like them dressed up, so this recipe does just that. Feel free to eliminate or shift any of the ingredients to match your diet.

2 pounds fresh brussels sprouts, halved

2 tablespoons extra-virgin olive oil

1 teaspoon sea salt

2 large apples *(Granny Smith or Red Delicious)*, chopped

⅓ cup dried cranberries

¾ cup chopped and toasted hazelnuts *or* pecans*

8 bacon strips, cooked and crumbled, divided *(optional)***

¼ cup local honey *or* maple syrup

⅓ cup apple cider vinegar

½ teaspoon coarsely ground black pepper

Substitutions:

*If nut free, omit the hazelnuts *or* pecans.

**If meat free, replace with Coconut Bacon *(page 157) or* Tempeh Bacon *(page 158).*

1) Preheat the oven to 400°F. Line a baking sheet with parchment paper.

2) Toss the brussels sprouts with the olive oil and sea salt and spread out on the prepared baking sheet. Roast for 20 minutes.

3) Transfer the brussels sprouts to a skillet over medium heat. Add the chopped apples, dried cranberries, and hazelnuts or pecans. Cook until the apples soften and the brussels sprouts crisp, about 5 to 8 minutes. Add the bacon.

4) In a bowl, whisk together the honey or syrup and vinegar. Pour over the brussels sprout mixture and warm through. Sprinkle with black pepper.

MY TIME IN MOROCCO INSPIRED THIS RECIPE, AS COUSCOUS IS A STAPLE on just about everyone's table. Making this dish grain free is what brings me joy, not because I believe grains are bad but because it's an opportunity to eat more veggies. Walnuts are the nut of choice because they support colon health, apricots add sweetness, and the cauliflower and carrots replace the couscous. I like to add different herbs and rotate my nuts each time I make this—you can also swap out the apricots for dried cranberries.

Chickpea Cauliflower "Couscous"

Makes 4 servings

½ cup dried apricots *(no sugar added)*, chopped

1 large head cauliflower, cut into florets

1 large carrot, chopped

2 tablespoons grass-fed butter *or* ghee, divided*

2 tablespoons extra-virgin olive oil, divided

1 medium onion, halved and thinly sliced

2 cloves garlic, minced

2½ cups fresh baby spinach

2 cups cooked chickpeas *or* 1 *(15.5 ounce)* can chickpeas, rinsed and drained

½ cup chopped, toasted walnuts

½ teaspoon sea salt

½ cup sliced scallions

Substitutions:

*If dairy free, replace with vegan butter.

1) Place the apricots in a small bowl. Cover with boiling water and let stand for 10 minutes or until plump; drain well.

2) Meanwhile, place the cauliflower in batches into a food processor. Cover and pulse each batch until crumbly and pieces resemble the texture of couscous. (Don't overpulse or the cauliflower will become mushy.)

3) Remove the cauliflower from the food processor and add the chopped carrots. Pulse until they also resemble the texture of couscous.

4) In an extra-large skillet, heat 1 tablespoon of the butter or ghee and 1 tablespoon of the olive oil over medium-high heat. Add the onion; cook and stir about 3 minutes or until tender and just starting to brown.

5) Add the garlic; cook and stir for 30 seconds more. Add the carrots, spread them out in the pan, and sauté for 4 minutes. Add the cauliflower to the pan, spreading in an even layer. Cook for about 8 minutes or until the cauliflower is golden brown, stirring occasionally. Spread it in an even layer after stirring.

6) Stir in the drained apricots, spinach, chickpeas, nuts, and sea salt. Cook and stir until combined. Stir in the remaining 1 tablespoon butter and scallions. Toss until the butter melts. Transfer to a serving bowl. Drizzle with the remaining 1 tablespoon of olive oil.

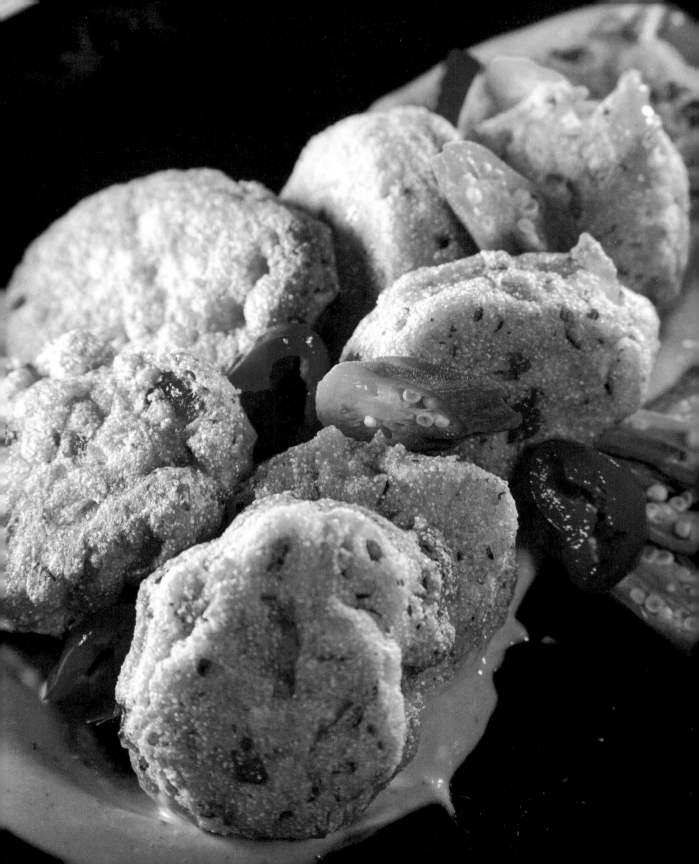

Okra Fritters

Makes 4 servings

WE HAVE ROWS AND rows of okra planted out on the farm. Once these flowers start turning to okra, we make OKRA EVERYTHING. You can't have a Southern cookbook without fritters, and okra makes 'em even betta'.

1 medium onion, roughly chopped

1 clove garlic

1 cup 1-to-1 gluten-free flour blend*

1 cup non-GMO cornmeal**

1 teaspoon sea salt

1 teaspoon baking powder

⅛ teaspoon cayenne pepper *or* 1 small jalapeño, de-seeded and chopped

1 egg *or* egg replacer equal to one egg

1 cup water

1 cup okra rounds

½ cup extra-virgin olive oil

Substitutions:

*If grain free, replace with coconut flour and double the egg.

**If corn free, replace with almond meal.

1) In a food processor, combine all the ingredients except for the okra and olive oil. Pulse until well blended. Transfer to a bowl and fold in the okra rounds.

2) Heat a skillet on medium-high heat and then add the olive oil. Once the oil is hot, drop medium-size spoonfuls of the okra mixture into the skillet. Cook each side for about 3 to 5 minutes until brown and crispy and then press to flatten.

3) Remove from the skillet and drain on a paper towel. Season with additional sea salt, if desired, to taste, and serve with a side of Quick Chipotle Aioli *(page 226)*.

REMINISCENT OF THE FALL, THESE carrots make a yummy side veggie to any main course, no matter the season.

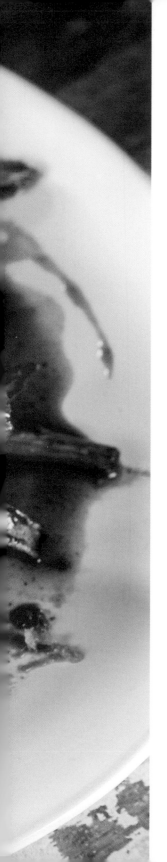

Orange Spice Carrots

Makes 4 servings

2 pounds medium carrots or baby carrots, cut into ¾-inch pieces

1 teaspoon extra-virgin olive oil

1 teaspoon sea salt, divided

2 tablespoons grass-fed butter *or* ghee*

½ cup fresh orange juice

½ cup coconut sugar**

¾ teaspoon ground cinnamon

¼ teaspoon ground nutmeg

1 tablespoon arrowroot powder *or* kuzu root

¼ cup cold water

½ teaspoon orange zest

Substitutions:

*If dairy free, replace with vegan butter.

**If watching sugar, omit it from this recipe.

1) Heat the oven to 400°F. Line a baking sheet with parchment paper.

2) Toss the carrots in the olive oil and sprinkle with ½ teaspoon of the sea salt. Spread the carrots on the prepared baking sheet and roast for 12 to 14 minutes.

3) Meanwhile, heat up a cast-iron pan over medium heat. Add the butter or ghee, orange juice, coconut sugar, cinnamon, nutmeg, remaining sea salt, arrowroot powder or kuzu root, and water.

4) Whisk until the sugar blends in and the sauce is smooth. Allow to simmer and reduce the liquid to a glaze-like consistency, for about 5 minutes, continuing to whisk to avoid burning.

5) Remove the carrots from the oven and toss with the glaze; sprinkle with orange zest.

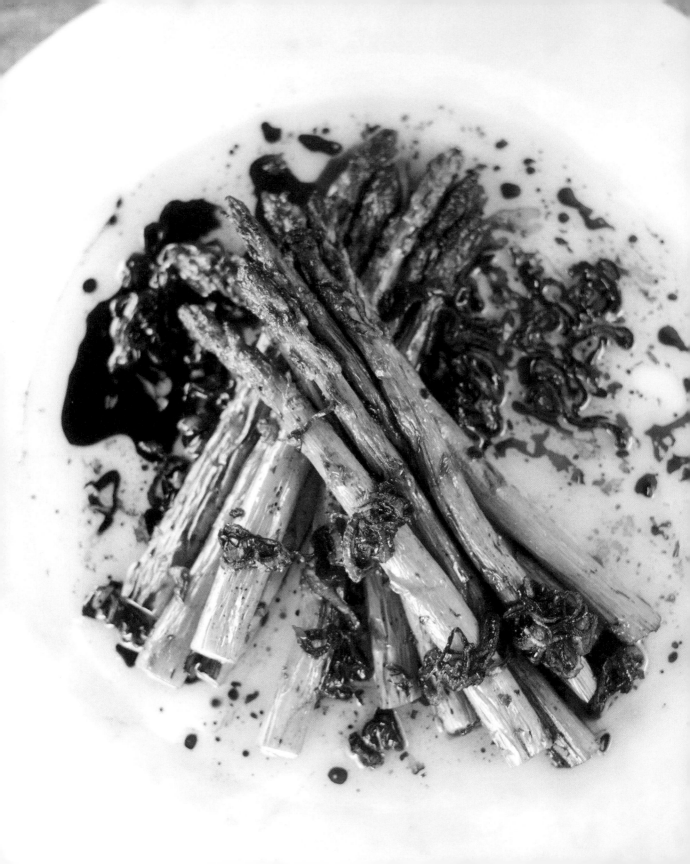

Roasted Asparagus with Shallot Vinaigrette

Makes 4 servings

SHALLOTS ARE SUPER GUT food. They are rich in flavonols and polyphenolic compounds. They also contain dietary fiber, protein, vitamin C, potassium, folate, vitamin B6, and vitamin A. Dang it, they are amazing! Asparagus, like other green vegetables, is high in antioxidants. These include vitamin E, vitamin C, and glutathione, as well as various flavonoids and polyphenols. Plus, asparagus feeds Bifidobacteria and Lactobacillus, both of which are important gut bacteria. These two bacteria are linked to strengthening the immune system. This combination of asparagus and shallots can be used in a number of dishes like salads, stir-fries, frittatas, omelets, and pastas.

1 pound fresh asparagus, trimmed

4 tablespoons extra-virgin olive oil, divided

½ teaspoon sea salt, divided

1 shallot, minced

1 tablespoon balsamic vinegar

¼ teaspoon black pepper

1) Preheat the oven to 425°F. Place the asparagus in a shallow baking pan or jelly-roll pan. Drizzle with 1 tablespoon of the oil and sprinkle with ¼ teaspoon of the sea salt; toss to coat.

2) Roast the asparagus for 8 minutes or until it's tender and lightly browned. Transfer to a serving dish.

3) Meanwhile, in a food processor or blender, add the remaining 3 tablespoons of the oil, the remaining sea salt, shallot, the vinegar, and the black pepper. Blend until well incorporated. Drizzle the dressing over the asparagus.

Tip: *When shopping for fresh asparagus, look for firm stems and tight, closed tips.*

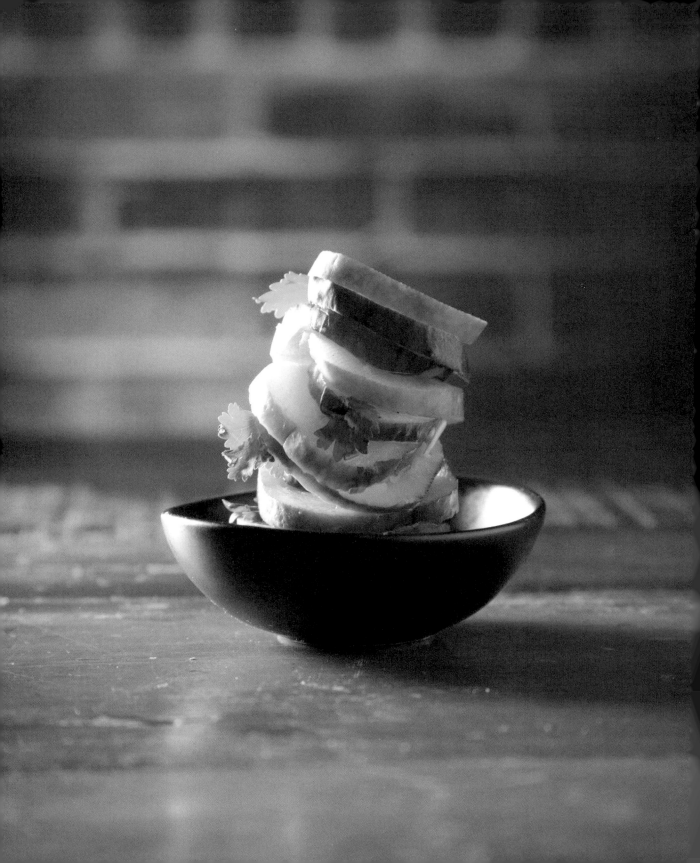

Homemade Cilantro Pickles

Makes 4 to 6 servings

THE SUMMER MONTHS
bring all the cucumbers to the
yard, and this means we get our
pickle on for the winter. In fact,
we pickle anything we have in
abundance. I appreciate homemade
pickles, and this recipe is easy
peasy. Plus, the apple cider vinegar
is a digestive aid. The cilantro,
cayenne, and onions are optional.
While I add them in for their
health benefits, you can leave
them out if they're not for you.
The pickles are still delicious
simple or dressed up!

¼ cup apple cider vinegar

2 medium cucumbers, sliced

½ red onion, thinly sliced *(optional)*

2 tablespoons chopped cilantro leaves *(optional)*

1 pinch cayenne pepper *(optional)*

1 tablespoon coconut sugar

½ teaspoon sea salt

1) Combine all the ingredients in a glass jar or bowl and
   cover in the refrigerator for a minimum of three hours.
   The longer they sit, the more pickled they become.

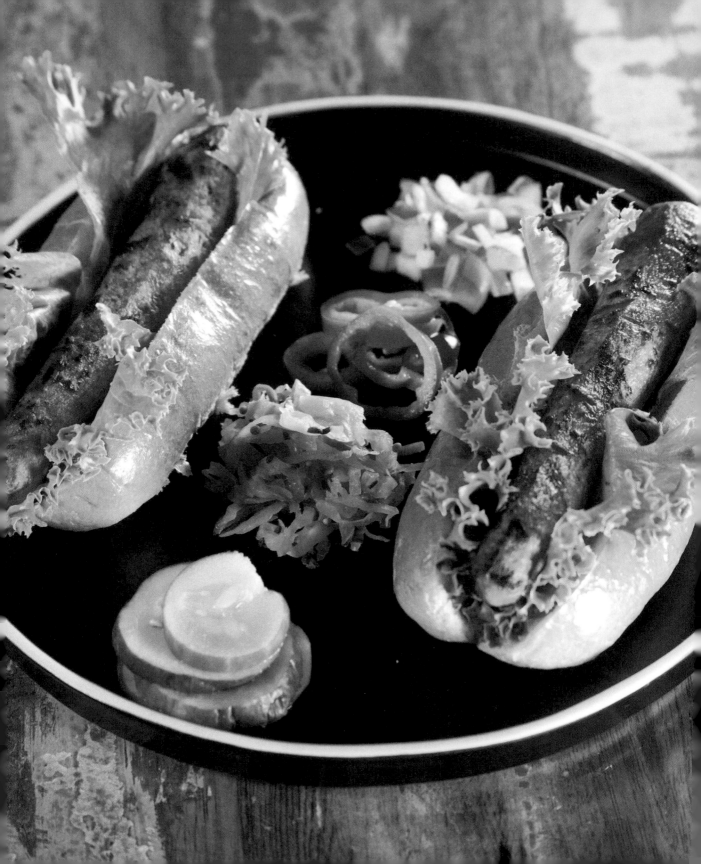

Carrot Wieners Pinewood-Style

Makes 8 servings

THIS IS PROBABLY THE MOST REQUESTED ITEM I'VE MADE ON TV.
Everyone wants a carrot wiener. Others think the idea is crazy, but once they try one, they are wowwwed!

1 cup Vegetable Broth *(page 121)*

1½ cups apple cider vinegar

2 tablespoons rice vinegar

2 tablespoons tamari *or* coconut aminos

½ teaspoon liquid smoke

1 tablespoon paprika

2 teaspoons mustard powder

½ teaspoon garlic powder

½ teaspoon ground coriander

¼ teaspoon black pepper

2 tablespoons extra-virgin olive oil

8 medium carrots, peeled with skinny ends trimmed and cut to the length of a hot dog bun

8 gluten-free hot dog buns *(such as Udi's)*

Toppings of choice

1) In a medium saucepan, mix together the broth, vinegars, tamari or coconut aminos, liquid smoke, paprika, mustard powder, garlic powder, coriander, and black pepper. Bring to a simmer. Let this marinade simmer for 5 minutes.

2) Meanwhile, toss the oil and the carrots together in a small roasting pan. Remove the marinade from the stovetop and pour it over the carrots. Cover and let it sit for at least 30 minutes and, preferably, up to 2 hours.

3) Preheat the oven to 425°F. Roast the carrots, covered, for 20 minutes. Uncover and stir them around, flipping them over, and roast for another 20 to 25 minutes. The carrots should be tender on the outside with a little bit of resistance in the center when pierced with a fork.

4) Place them on the buns and serve with a variety of traditional hot dog toppings.

Pickled Carmen Peppers

Makes 2 cups

WE GROW ALL KINDS OF peppers, sweet and spicy. My favorites are the red Carmen Italian sweet peppers. They are crazy sweet and the perfect amount of crisp goodness. We pickle them and then run 'em through the canner so we can top salads, side dishes, and soups throughout the winter until they return again in the summer. You can use any type of pepper you like for this recipe.

1 cup apple cider vinegar

1 cup water

½ cup coconut sugar

1 teaspoon sea salt

6 to 9 Carmen peppers, stems removed, thinly sliced into rounds *(about 3 cups)*

1) In a small saucepan over high heat, combine the apple cider vinegar, water, coconut sugar, and sea salt, stirring until the salt and sugar dissolve.

2) Remove the saucepan from the heat and add the sliced peppers. Stir for about 15 seconds, as the peppers soften. The peppers should become mostly submerged in the liquid.

3) Allow the mixture to cool to room temperature. Pour the peppers into a jar and drain the excess liquid; the peppers should just be covered in liquid; store in the fridge.

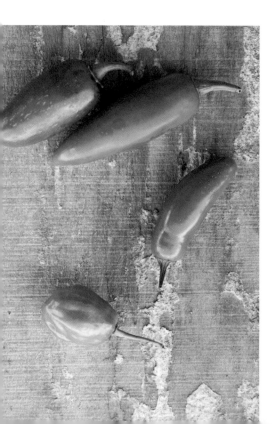

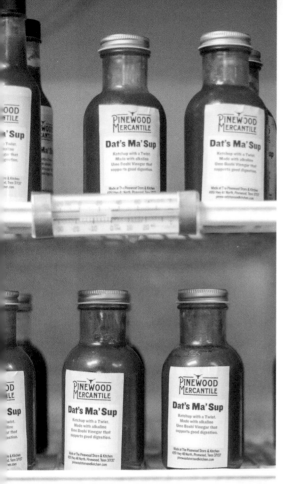
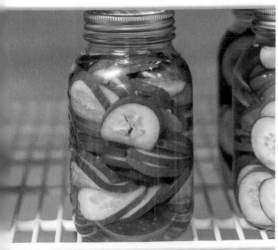
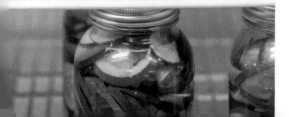

Dips, Spreads, Sauces, Faux Cheez & More

It's the simple things that inspire our tables in Pinewood Kitchen, and the showstoppers are often the condiments. Serving homemade ketchup, mayo, ranch dressing, and chipotle aioli is how we show off and show out. Bringing these delicious recipes to your table will take the guilt away and add a smile to everyone who dips.

I'M A HUMMUS LOVER, AND HARISSA IS A GUT-SUPPORTING CONDIMENT that I keep both in my Pinewood Kitchen and home kitchen. Miso is the probiotic that all the other prebiotic foods in this recipe need.

Cauliflower & Harissa Probiotic Hummus

Makes 4 servings

2 cups cauliflower florets

2 cups cooked chickpeas *or*
1 *(15.5-ounce)* can chickpeas,
rinsed and drained

2 tablespoons Homemade Harissa
Paste *(page 209)**

¼ cup tahini

¼ cup freshly squeezed lemon juice

¼ cup extra-virgin olive oil

½ teaspoon miso

½ teaspoon sea salt

¼ teaspoon paprika

1 clove garlic, minced

1 tablespoon chopped fresh parsley

Dippers

Sliced red peppers

Broccoli florets

Carrot sticks

Sliced radishes

Garden vegetables of choice

Substitutions

*If short on time, replace with store-bought harissa paste.

1) In a medium saucepan over medium heat, add the cauliflower florets and enough water to cover the cauliflower only partway. Cover the pan and allow the water to boil. Steam for approximately 10 minutes or until tender; drain. Transfer the cauliflower to a bowl of ice water until cool; drain well.

2) In a food processor, combine the cauliflower, chickpeas, harissa paste, tahini, lemon juice, olive oil, miso, sea salt, paprika, and garlic. Cover and blend until smooth, about 4 minutes, stopping and scraping the sides as necessary.

3) Transfer the hummus to a small serving bowl. Sprinkle with the parsley. If desired, swirl additional harissa paste on top of the hummus just before serving. Serve with vegetable dippers of choice.

Pumpkin Seed Dip

Makes about 2¼ cups

I'M ALWAYS thinking about what to serve my friends who can't have nuts. This dip is a crowd-pleaser regardless of whether you can or can't eat nuts. If you have digestive issues and can't eat seeds, this is a great alternative that's as delicious as it is nutritious.

1½ cups pumpkin seeds

2 medium Roma tomatoes

¼ medium white onion, sliced

1 habanero *or* 2 jalapeños *or* serrano peppers

1 tablespoon extra-virgin olive oil

3 tablespoons orange juice

2 cloves garlic, minced

½ teaspoon sea salt

1 tablespoon finely chopped fresh chives

1 tablespoon finely chopped fresh cilantro

¼ cup chopped tomatoes *(optional)*

1 recipe Baked Tortilla Chips/Tostadas *(page 212)**

Substitutions:

*If short on time, use high-quality store-bought tostadas made from corn *or* almond meal.

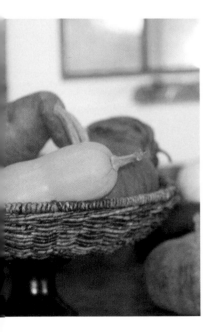

1) Preheat the oven to 350°F. Spread the pumpkin seeds on a large baking sheet. Bake for 8 minutes or until toasted. Spread the seeds on parchment paper to cool. Increase the oven temperature to 450°F.

2) Place the whole tomatoes, onion, and pepper in a baking pan. Drizzle with oil; toss to coat. Roast for 10 to 12 minutes or until tender and lightly charred; cool slightly.

3) Core the tomatoes and remove the skins. Wearing kitchen gloves, remove the stem and seeds from the pepper. Remove and discard the large dry pieces of charred tomato skin but not all of it.

4) Place the pumpkin seeds in a food processor; process until ground. Add the roasted tomatoes, onions, and peppers, orange juice, garlic, and sea salt; process until nearly smooth. Stir in the chives and cilantro.

5) If desired, top with additional tomatoes. Serve with baked tostadas.

Homemade Harissa Paste

Makes 4 servings

THE INGREDIENTS in harissa are all about supporting the gut. Harissa is a traditional condiment that's loaded with immune-supporting caraway seeds, coriander, cumin, garlic, and chilis—all the flavorful ingredients you want in a condiment.

4 ounces dried ancho *and/or* pasilla peppers*

½ teaspoon caraway seeds

½ teaspoon coriander seeds

½ teaspoon cumin seeds

5 cloves garlic, peeled

3 tablespoons extra-virgin olive oil

2 tablespoons lemon juice

1 teaspoon kosher sea salt

3 to 4 tablespoons water

Substitutions:

*If avoiding spicy food, replace with sweet red bell peppers.

1) Place the dried chili peppers in a large bowl. Pour enough boiling water over the peppers to cover; let stand for 20 minutes.

2) In a small skillet over medium heat, heat the caraway, coriander, and cumin seeds for 2 minutes or until toasted and aromatic, shaking the skillet occasionally. Remove the seeds from the skillet; let cool. Grind the seeds in a spice grinder or crush with a mortar and pestle.

3) Drain the peppers. Wear plastic or rubber gloves to remove the stems, seeds, and membranes from the peppers. In a food processor or blender, combine the peppers, ground or crushed seeds, garlic, olive oil, lemon juice, and sea salt. Cover and pulse until smooth, adding water, as needed, to reach a smooth consistency. Transfer to a jar with a lid, and store in the fridge.

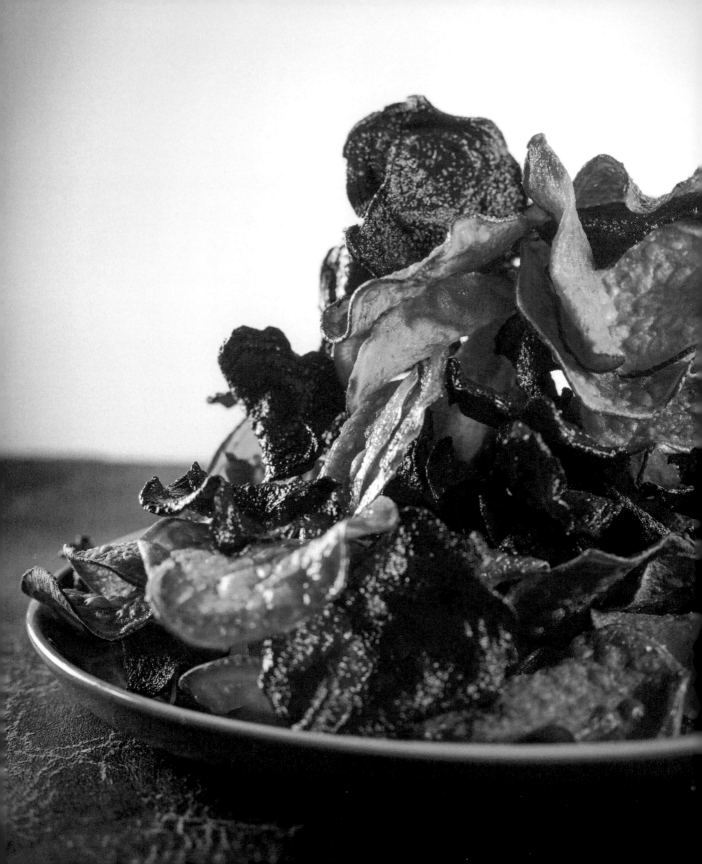

Baked Sweet Potato and Beet Chips

Makes 4 servings

I'M A CHIP-EATING GIRL.
Hand me a bag of potato chips and I'm happy. But potato chips are not the best choice. This recipe is a great substitute and serves as a wonderful appetizer or party snack. This is a good corn chip replacement for those avoiding corn and grains. These are delicious with fresh guacamole or any dip you like.

Nonstick coconut oil cooking spray

2 large sweet potatoes, peeled

2 large beets, trimmed and peeled

½ teaspoon sea salt

¼ teaspoon black pepper

¼ teaspoon ground ancho chile pepper

1) Preheat the oven to 375°F. Lightly coat two baking sheets with coconut oil cooking spray.

2) Using a mandoline slicer, cut the potatoes and beets into slices about one-sixteenth of an inch thick. Sandwich the beet slices between paper towels and press firmly to remove the excess moisture. (There's no need to blot the sweet potatoes.)

3) Arrange the slices on the prepared baking sheets. Coat the slices with cooking spray and sprinkle with sea salt, black pepper, and chile pepper.

4) Bake for 10 minutes. Remove from the oven and let stand for 5 minutes. Return to the oven and bake for 4 to 8 more minutes, checking the chips every minute and then removing them when the center of the chips appears dry. Transfer to paper towels and cool for 5 minutes.

Baked Tortilla Chips/Tostadas

Makes 64 chips or 8 tostadas

I LOVE TORTILLAS,

and I would say my excess guilty
pleasure is eating dry, crunchy
snacks. Making my own dry,
crunchy snacks is how I keep my
gut healthy by avoiding processed
foods.

**8 *(6-inch)* corn *and/or* almond meal tortillas *or* Cassava
Tortillas *(page 240)***

1) Preheat the oven to 350°F. Cut tortilla into eight wedges.
   If making tostadas, do not cut them—bake them whole.

2) Spread the wedges or whole tortillas on two large baking
   sheets; sprinkle lightly with sea salt.

3) Bake for 12 to 15 minutes or until crisp and light brown.

Basic Mayo

Makes about 1 cup

MAKE YOUR OWN MAYO

when you can—it's not
complicated, and then you
know exactly what's in it.
Most store-bought mayo
contains soybean oil and tons
of additives. This recipe is
quick and easy. In Pinewood,
we use our own farm-fresh
eggs.

1 cup extra-virgin olive oil

1 egg yolk

2 teaspoons champagne vinegar

¼ teaspoon sea salt

2 teaspoons water

1) Pour the olive oil in a glass measuring cup or pitcher that you
   can easily handle with one hand while whisking with the other.

2) In a medium nonreactive bowl (such as stainless steel or glass),
   whisk the egg yolk vigorously while adding the oil drop by drop.
   Incorporate each drop before adding the next. As the mixture
   thickens and emulsifies, begin adding the remaining oil in a
   slow, steady stream, continuing to whisk vigorously, until you
   have added all the oil. The mixture should be thick and glossy.

3) Whisk in the vinegar, sea salt, and water until fully incorporated.
   Store in the fridge and briefly whisk before using.

Vegan Mayo

Makes about 1½ cups

WE ARE MINDFUL OF EGG allergies in Pinewood Kitchen, and we also want to be able to accommodate vegan guests. It's important to have mayo-based foods that can support them. Plus, finding vegan mayo in the store that isn't made with soybean oil is tough.

1 cup avocado oil

½ cup unsweetened oat milk *or* soy milk

1 tablespoon extra-virgin olive oil

½ teaspoon sea salt

2 teaspoons white vinegar

1 tablespoon maple syrup *(optional)*

1) Place all the ingredients in a bowl. Using an immersion or handheld blender, blend until creamy.

Cashew Sour Cream

Makes about 1 cup

THIS RICH AND CREAMY SOUR cream can be folded into all kinds of recipes that call for sour cream or used as a topper on tacos.

½ cup raw cashews

¾ cup water

2 tablespoons fresh lemon juice

2 teaspoons apple cider vinegar

½ teaspoon sea salt

1) Soak the cashews overnight, and rinse well or boil them for 15 to 20 minutes; strain the liquid.

2) In a food processor or high-speed blender, combine all the ingredients. Blend on high until super smooth. Stop occasionally to scrape down the sides of the blender. Add a little more water as needed for a smoother consistency. Transfer to a dish with a cover, and store in the fridge.

Coconut Sour Cream

Makes about 1 cup

I LOVE SOUR CREAM, BUT WHEN
I had gut issues it didn't love me back! This is a delicious sour cream replacement that will make you rejoice if you are missing that creamy goodness on top of your chili, tacos, or nachos. It's pure yum! Lots of folks have nut allergies and can't have cashew sour cream. By using coconut milk, this is a wonderful alternative. Just make sure the coconut milk has not been processed in a facility that processes nuts if you are cooking for someone with severe nut allergies.

1 can full-fat coconut milk, chilled overnight

2 tablespoons lemon juice

¼ teaspoon apple cider vinegar

⅛ teaspoon sea salt

1) Open the can of coconut milk with the can upside down; drain off the liquid, which is coconut water, and save for other uses.

2) Scrape the thick coconut cream directly into a blender or food processor.

3) Add the remaining ingredients and blend until smooth and creamy. Transfer to a dish with a cover and store in the fridge.

Creamy Cashew Spread

Makes about 1 cup

THIS YUMMY SPREAD IS a great cream cheese replacement.

1 cup raw cashews

2 tablespoons lemon juice

1 tablespoon tahini

½ teaspoon sea salt

½ teaspoon black pepper

2 tablespoons minced fresh herbs, such as basil, parsley, *or* oregano *(optional)*

Assorted gluten-free bread, toast, *and/or* crackers

1) Rinse the cashews and place them in a medium bowl. Cover with water by at least 2 inches; soak for 4 hours or overnight. Drain the cashews, reserving the soaking water.

2) In a food processor or blender, combine the cashews, 2 tablespoons of the reserved water, lemon juice, tahini, sea salt, and black pepper; process for several minutes or until smooth. Add additional water, 1 tablespoon at a time, until the desired consistency is reached.

3) Cover and refrigerate until ready to serve. Stir in herbs, if desired, just before serving. Serve with assorted bread, toasts, and/or crackers.

Tip: *If you are not happy with how your cheese turned out, blame it on the agar flakes. It's best to measure these by weight instead of volume because flake cuts differ from brand to brand.*

Rockin' Faux Cheddar

Makes 4 cups

CAN'T HAVE nachos without the cheese, baby! I use this bettah cheddah to whip up my childhood favorites, like good ole mac and cheese and grilled cheese, and as a sauce over peas. Made with cashews, this cheez is not only antioxidant rich but it is also packed full of the same heart-healthy fat found in olive oil.

1¼ cups raw cashews

½ cup nutritional yeast

2 teaspoons onion powder

2 teaspoons sea salt

1 teaspoon garlic powder

⅛ teaspoon ground white pepper

3½ cups unsweetened soymilk *or* other dairy-free milk

2 ounces agar flakes *(about 1 cup)*

½ cup extra-virgin olive oil

¼ cup yellow miso

2 tablespoons freshly squeezed lemon juice

1) Rinse the cashews and place them in a medium bowl. Cover with water by at least 2 inches; soak 4 hours or overnight. Drain the cashews, reserving the soaking water.

2) In a food processor, finely grind the cashews using the pulse button, without allowing them to turn into paste. Add in the yeast, onion powder, sea salt, garlic powder, and white pepper. Pulse a few more times to blend. Set aside in the food processor.

3) In a heavy saucepan, combine the nondairy milk, agar, and oil and bring to a simmer over high heat. Decrease the heat to medium-low and cover and simmer. Stir occasionally for 10 minutes or until the agar is dissolved.

4) With the food processor running, pour the soymilk mixture through the feed tube into the cashew mixture. Blend for 2 minutes, and then add in the miso and lemon juice.

5) Use immediately as melted cheez, or store covered in the fridge and remelt the "cheez" in a saucepan, adding more milk for a thinner consistency. For grated or sliced cheez, refrigerate for 4 hours or until firm, and then grate or slice.

THIS SAUCE IS EXCELLENT FOR THOSE FOLKS AVOIDING NIGHTSHADES AND HISTAMINES.
It's so easy to make as you just put it all in a pot and puree. You can also doctor it up with even more herbs!
It's basically like making marinara sauce without the tomatoes. This is great over gluten-free pasta.

Tomato-Free Marinara Sauce

Makes 4 to 6 servings

FOR THE BASE:

6 carrots, cut in 2-inch pieces

1 small beet, quartered

1 large onion

1 stalk celery, sliced

3 cloves garlic

3 cups water

FOR THE FLAVOR:

1 to 2 teaspoons extra-virgin olive oil

3 cloves garlic, minced

1 teaspoon chopped fresh basil

1 teaspoon chopped fresh oregano

1 bay leaf

¼ cup minced fresh Italian parsley

1 cup mushrooms of choice, sliced *or* chopped *(optional)*

2 tablespoons miso *or* tamari

1 teaspoon umeboshi vinegar*

2 heaping tablespoons kuzu root, dissolved in ½ cup cool water

*For this, you gotta use your taste buds to get it right; this ingredient is key to bringing in that tangy tomato flavor.

1) In a large pot, combine the carrots, beet, onion, celery, garlic, and water. Boil until the veggies are super soft—about 30 minutes. Allow to cool.

2) Transfer the veggies to a blender or use an immersion blender in the pot. Blend until you achieve the texture of tomato sauce. Add more water if needed. Set aside.

3) Heat the oil in a saucepan. Sauté the garlic, onion, and herbs for 5 minutes. Add the mushrooms (if using, to impart a meaty texture), and sauté for 10 more minutes. Add the sauce to the pan and bring to a boil.

4) Cover and simmer for 1 hour—just like real sauce. The longer it cooks together, the better. Add the miso or tamari and the vinegar. Add the kuzu root, stirring until thick and shiny. Remove the bay leaf before serving.

Kuzu Mushroom Gravy

Makes about 2 cups

I AM A GRAVY-LOVING woman and so are most folks in Pinewood. This recipe, served on top of mashed potatoes or polenta, is pure comfort food with a healing twist.

2 tablespoons extra-virgin olive oil

½ onion, chopped fine

2 cloves garlic, minced

1 cup fresh shiitake mushrooms

2 tablespoons tamari *or* coconut aminos

2 cups water *or* broth of choice

1 tablespoon miso

2 tablespoons kuzu root diluted in 4 tablespoons cold water

1) Heat a small pot over medium-low; add the olive oil, onion, garlic, mushrooms, tamari or coconut aminos, and the water or broth. Bring to a strong simmer. Add the miso paste and whisk.

2) Add the diluted kuzu root, whisking constantly to avoid lumps. Remove from the heat once it has thickened to your liking.

The Incredible Kuzu Root

I fell hard for this edible root. Kuzu is widely used in Asian cooking as a thickener. It is very low in calories, contains no fat, and is an easily digestible source of complex carbohydrates—only 8 grams per serving. Kuzu root is so strong that it can grow through concrete and rock!

When eaten, it lends its strength to healing the intestinal lining in our bodies. Our intestines are the roots of our bodies, and **all** health issues stem from weakened intestinal walls because that is where the body receives nutrition. If the tissue there is damaged, our bodies can't get the nutrition we need.

Eating root vegetables brings "core" strength and aids in balancing our health. Ancestral people claim that if the intestinal wall is weak, then kuzu will strengthen it. If the wall is too tough, kuzu will soften it. Kuzu is a natural ulcerative Band-Aid, easing intestinal sores while the body heals.

Pinewood Pepper Sauce

Makes about 3 cups

WHEN IT PEPPERS, IT
pours—meaning we grow an insane amount of peppers, and not wasting them is a big goal of ours in Pinewood Kitchen. Folks love hot sauce, and creating one without additives, preservatives, or corn syrup is important to me. This pepper sauce is excellent added to soup or served with our crispy fried fish.

2 cups hot peppers of choice

½ cup coconut sugar*

4 cups apple cider vinegar

1 cup water

4 cloves garlic, smashed

Substitutions:

*If watching sugar, use an equivalent amount of stevia (page 51).

1) Using a sharp knife, poke slits in each pepper to allow the peppers to absorb the vinegar.

2) In a stainless steel soup pot over medium-high heat, combine all the ingredients, and bring to a rolling boil.

3) Lower the heat to simmer and cook for 15 minutes. Remove from the heat and allow the mixture to steep and then cool for 20 minutes.

4) Pour into a blender and puree. Use as is for a thicker sauce or run it through a sieve for a thinner sauce.

5) Transfer to a jar or glass bottle with a lid and store in the fridge.

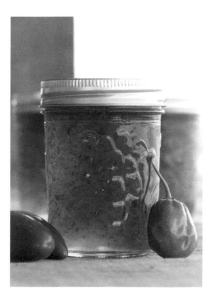

WE SERVE THIS WITH MANY
different dishes in Pinewood and always
with our veggie and grain bowls.

Sweet Chili Sauce

Makes about 1¾ cups

½ cup rice vinegar

¾ cup water

½ cup plus 2 tablespoons coconut sugar*

5 garlic cloves, crushed

1 tablespoon tamari *or* coconut aminos

½ tablespoon fish sauce *(optional)*

½ teaspoon cayenne pepper

2½ tablespoons sambal oelek chili paste *or* sriracha

4 teaspoons arrowroot powder *or* kuzu root

2 tablespoons water

Substitutions:

*If watching sugar, use an equivalent amount of stevia *(page 51)*.

1) In a large saucepan over medium heat, add the vinegar, water, sugar, garlic, tamari or coconut aminos, fish sauce, and cayenne pepper. Stir constantly to dissolve the sugar. Increase the heat to medium high and bring to a boil. Let it simmer for about 5 minutes.

2) Add the chili paste or sriracha and mix.

3) In a small dish, dilute the arrowroot powder or kuzu root in the water until it's smooth and add to the sauce.

4) While stirring frequently to prevent the sauce from burning at the bottom, simmer the sauce for a few more minutes until it thickens into a ketchup-like consistency. The sauce will thicken more as it cools. If it becomes too thick, add a little water to thin it. Once cooled, store in a glass jar in the fridge.

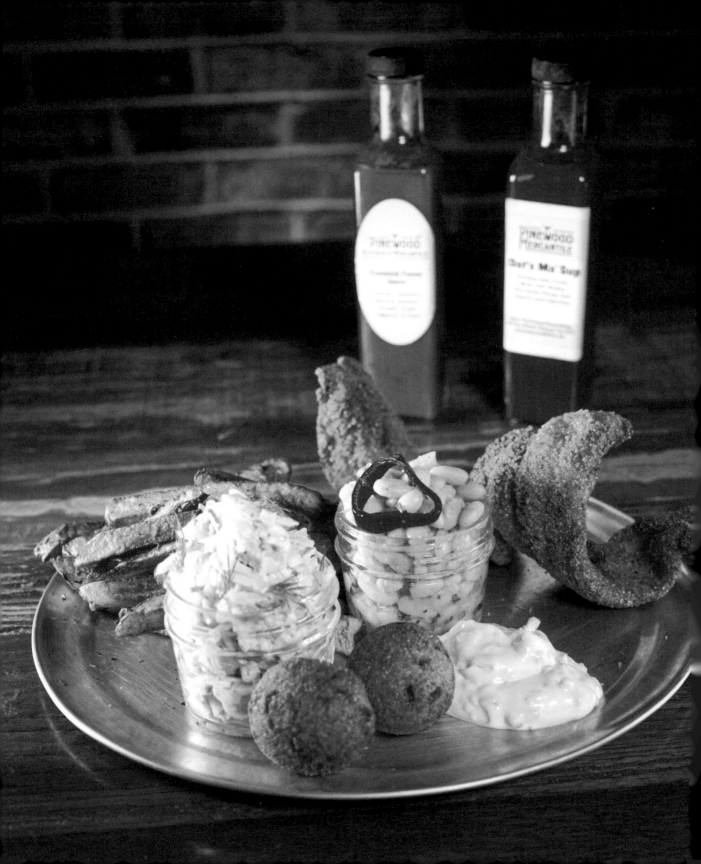

Dat's Ma Sup Ketchup

Makes 3 cups

WE CAN'T KEEP THIS
stuff in stock in the
mercantile, and we have
people who hate ketchup but
love ours. Made with apple
cider vinegar and umeboshi
vinegar, this ketchup has
great flavor and helps with
acid reflux because it serves
as a digestive aid.

2 cups homemade *or* canned tomato sauce

½ cup apple cider vinegar

¼ cup umeboshi vinegar

1 teaspoon crushed fresh garlic *or* garlic powder

½ cup local honey *or* coconut sugar*

Substitutions:

*If watching sugar, use an equivalent amount of stevia
(page 51).

1) In a blender, combine all the ingredients. Blend until
   smooth. Scraping the sides of the blender, transfer the
   ketchup to a glass jar with a lid. Store in the fridge.

Quick Chipotle Aioli

Makes about 1 cup

I LOVE TO DIP, AND I LOVE to dip into something spicy. Chipotle aioli is easy to make and it adds a delicious zing to everything. Add it to a falafel burger and it's a hit!

1 cup Vegan Mayo *(page 213) or* Basic Mayo *(page 212)*

2 tablespoons finely chopped chives

2 cloves garlic, minced

1 teaspoon fresh lime juice

2 teaspoons ground chipotle *or* 2 chipotles from a 7-ounce tin of chipotle pepper in adobo sauce

1 teaspoon adobo sauce

Sea salt *(to taste)*

1) In a blender, combine all the ingredients. Blend until smooth and creamy. Scraping the sides of the blender, transfer the aioli to a glass bowl for serving.

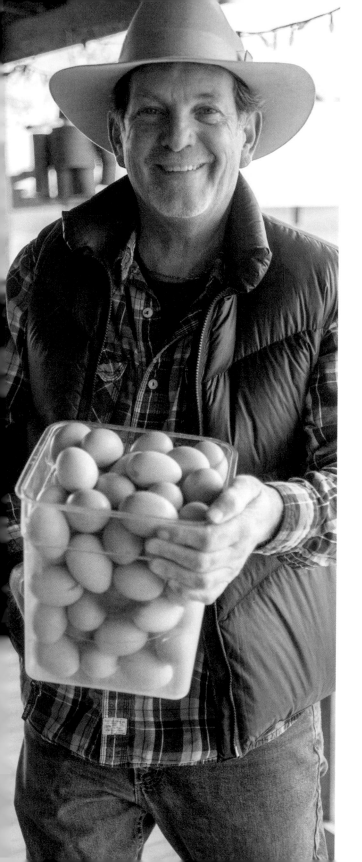

Farmhouse Breakfast Favorites

I'm not a major breakfast eater as I do like to practice intermittent fasting. I've been doing so for about ten years because it was recommended to me as a way to give my weakened intestines a break. I do, however, start my day with a smoothie or a warm bowl of leftover soup. But, on the weekends when I have time with the kids, or I am running Pinewood Kitchen's brunch, I have some favorites, and these are just a few.

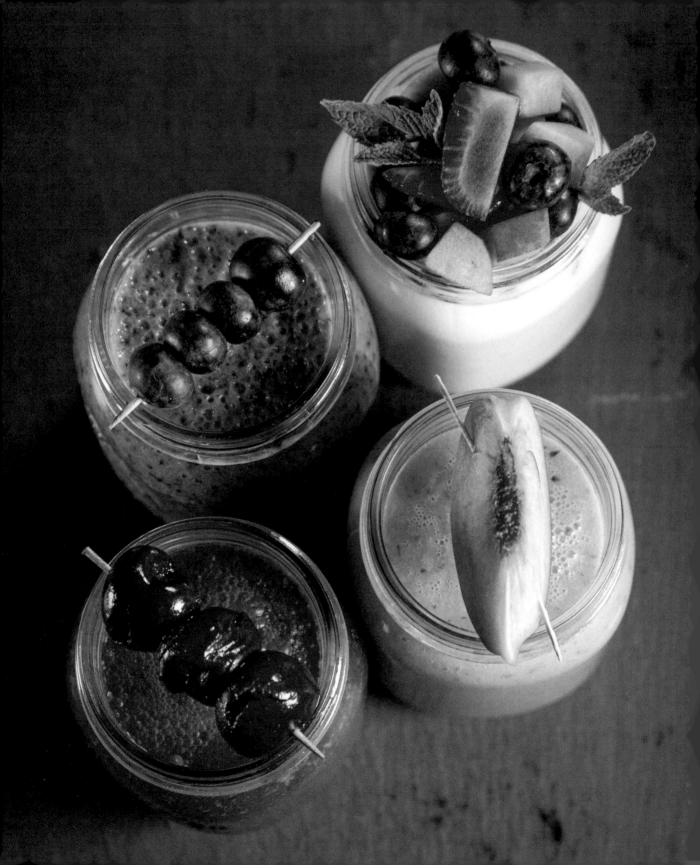

Black Forest Smoothie

Makes 2 servings

THIS SMOOTHIE IS DECADENT and rich. If it's too thick for your liking, add more liquid. I like my smoothies thick because many times they are my meal replacements.

1 cup frozen cherries

1 cup tart cherry juice

½ medium ripe avocado

½ frozen banana

3 tablespoons unsweetened cocoa powder

2 tablespoons unsweetened sunflower seed butter *or* almond butter

2 cups water

Pinch sea salt

1 scoop lion's mane mushroom powder

1 scoop maca powder

1 scoop greens powder

1) Place the ingredients in a blender in the order listed. Blend on high until creamy and smooth. Serve immediately.

Here's the Scoop with a "Scoop"

Usually, powders come with a handy scooper that measures out a single serving. If you're not sure, check the suggested serving size on the label of your product.

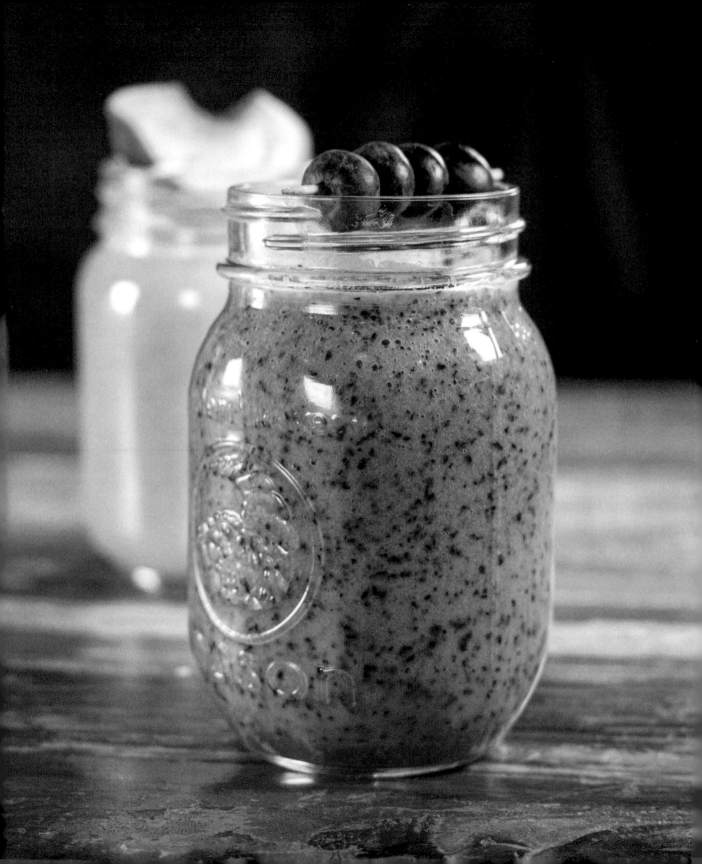

Blueberry Smoothie

Makes 2 servings

THIS IS MY GO-TO
smoothie. I always have a bag of frozen cranberries and organic frozen blueberries on hand, and during blueberry season in Pinewood, I use fresh blueberries. Loaded with antioxidants and prebiotic fiber, this is the one recipe I recommend adding to your weekly groove as it's easy and delish.

½ cup organic or wild blueberries

½ cup whole frozen cranberries

1 tablespoon dairy-free yogurt

1 scoop organic dairy-free vanilla protein powder *or* 2 tablespoons nut butter *or* seed butter

¼ cup pomegranate juice

1 cup flax milk

2 cups water

1 scoop mushroom powder of choice

1 scoop maca powder

1 scoop greens powder

1) Place the ingredients in a blender in the order listed. Blend on high until creamy and smooth. Serve immediately.

Blueberry Peach Smoothie

Makes 2 servings

THERE'S NOTHING MORE
Southern than peaches, and adding them to my smoothie is a great way to lighten and brighten my day. Toss in blueberries and pomegranate juice, and it's an antioxidant palooza.

½ cup organic *or* wild blueberries

¼ cup whole frozen cranberries

½ cup frozen peaches

1 cup flax milk

2 cups water

¼ cup pomegranate juice

1 scoop organic dairy-free vanilla protein powder *or* 2 tablespoons nut butter or seed butter

1 scoop mushroom powder of choice

1 scoop maca powder

1 scoop greens powder

1) Place the ingredients in a blender in the order listed. Blend on high until creamy and smooth. Serve immediately.

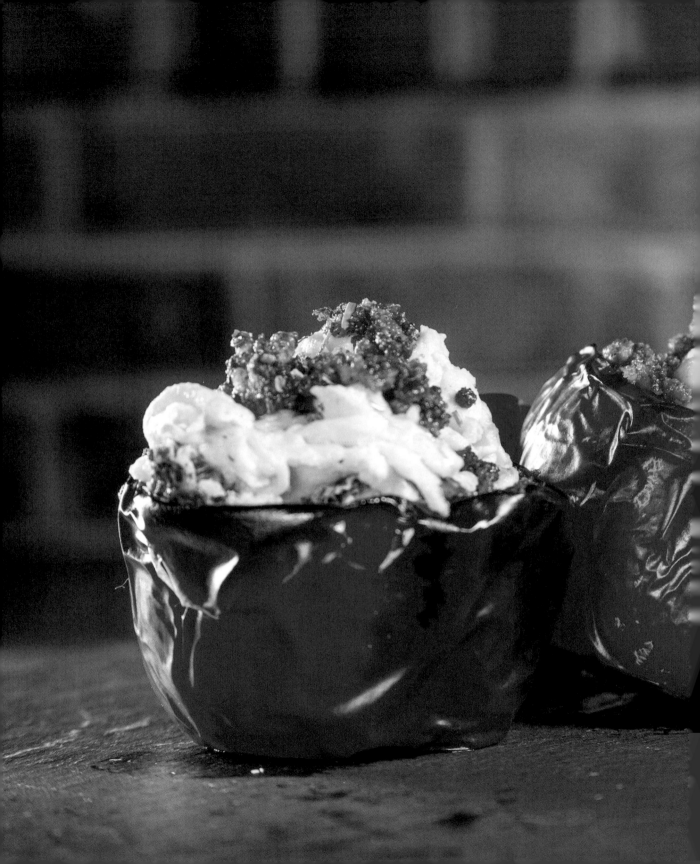

Farm Fresh Egg and Sausage Stuffed Bell Peppers

Makes 2 to 4 servings

THIS IS A GREAT brunch recipe that looks beautiful on the plate. In Pinewood, we make our own sausage with a touch of fennel. The reason for the fennel is it's a digestive aid and lends a complementary flavor to pork. I make my sausage ahead of time and store it in the fridge until I'm ready to make breakfast or brunch. You can use any type of sausage you'd like.

4 medium red or yellow bell peppers, halved and seeded

6 large eggs

½ cup nondairy milk

1 teaspoon sea salt

¼ teaspoon black pepper

¼ cup chopped scallions, plus more for garnish

1 cup cooked and crumbled pork, turkey, *or* vegan sausage

1) Preheat the oven to 350°F.

2) Line a baking sheet or dish with parchment paper and arrange the peppers on top, cavity side up.

3) In a medium bowl, whisk together the eggs, milk, salt, and black pepper. Stir in the scallions and sausage.

4) Pour the mixture evenly into the bell pepper halves and bake for 45 minutes.

5) Garnish with fresh scallions. Serve alongside a small mixed greens salad, if desired.

Tip: *It's best to gather all of your ingredients and have them on hand and measured out before you begin a recipe. This simplifies your flow in the kitchen.*

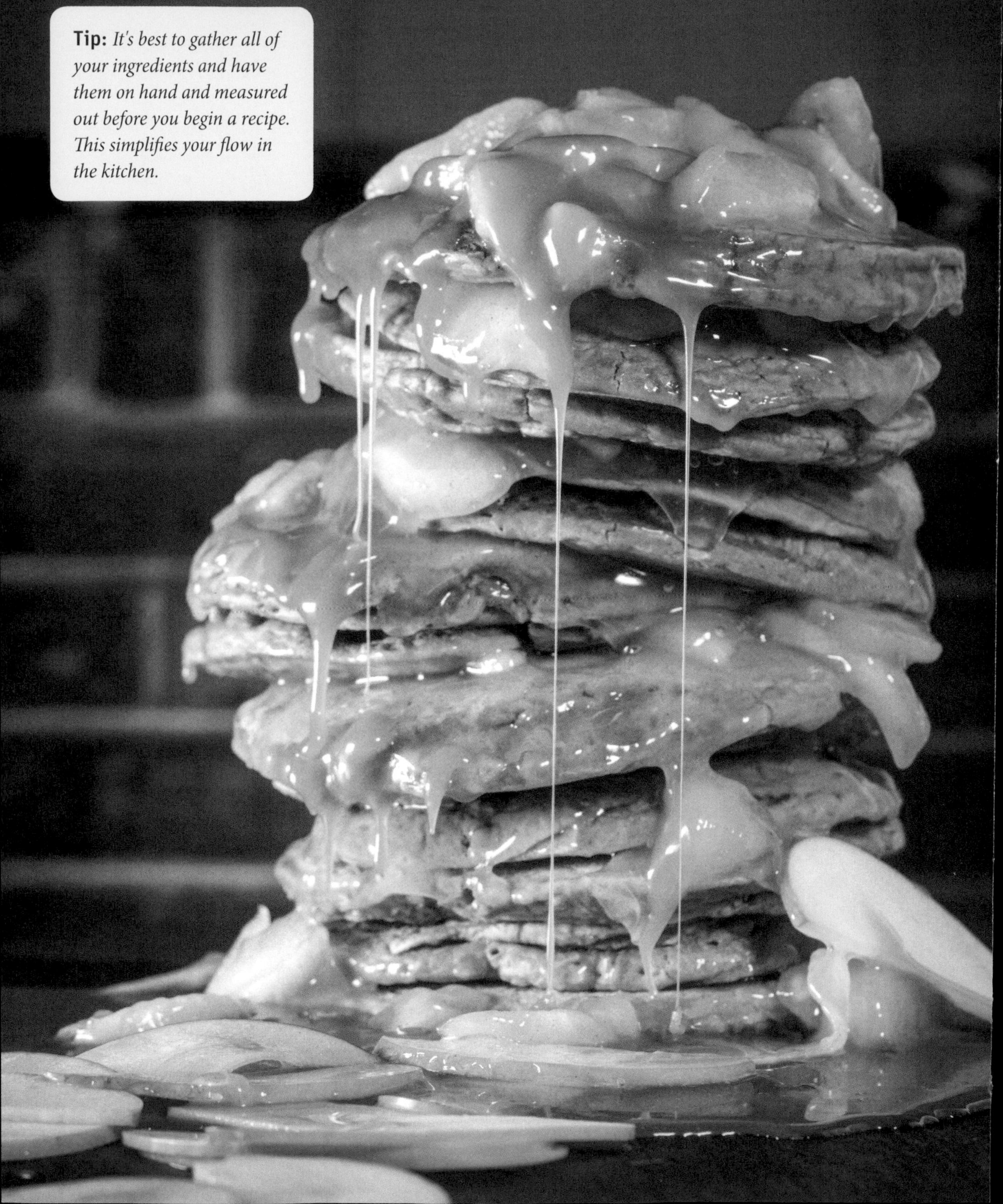

Caramel Apple Buckwheat Pancakes

Makes 4 servings

WET INGREDIENTS:

1 tablespoon ground flaxseeds

3 tablespoons water

1¼ cups plus 2 tablespoons almond milk

2 tablespoons melted coconut oil

1 cup finely chopped Granny Smith *or* Red Delicious apples

DRY INGREDIENTS:

1¾ cups buckwheat flour

2 teaspoons baking powder

2 tablespoons coconut sugar

¼ teaspoon fine sea salt

2 teaspoons ground cinnamon

FOR THE COCONUT CARAMEL APPLES:

3 teaspoons coconut oil

4 tablespoons coconut sugar

1 teaspoon ground cinnamon

2 tablespoons water

Granny Smith apple *or* Red Delicious, peeled and cut into wedges

1) In a medium bowl, combine the flaxseeds and 3 tablespoons of the water to make a "flax egg." Let it rest for 5 minutes.

2) In a separate medium bowl, combine all the dry ingredients, sifting or whisking them together.

3) In the medium bowl with the flax egg, add 1¼ cups of the almond milk.

4) Gently fold the wet mixture into the dry mixture. Be careful not to overmix the batter. Let the pancake batter rest for 15 minutes. This allows all the ingredients to work together so your pancakes will rise a little bit. Once the batter has rested, fold in the additional 2 tablespoons of almond milk, the 2 tablespoons of coconut oil, and the chopped apple.

5) Place a few drops of coconut oil on a good quality non-stick frying pan over low-medium heat and spread it in the pan using a paper towel. This is all the oil you will need. Between pancakes, carefully rub the same paper towel on the pan.

6) Pour ¼ cup of the batter on the heated pan. Cook for 2 to 3 minutes until bubbles start popping on the surface. Flip the pancake over and cook for about 2 more minutes. Continue with the remaining batter.

7) To make the caramel apples, melt the 3 teaspoons of coconut oil, and add the coconut sugar, cinnamon, and the 2 tablespoons of water. Mix together, allowing the ingredients to combine into a smooth caramel sauce. Add the apple wedges and cook until soft and warm.

8) Serve the caramel apples over the pancakes and enjoy!

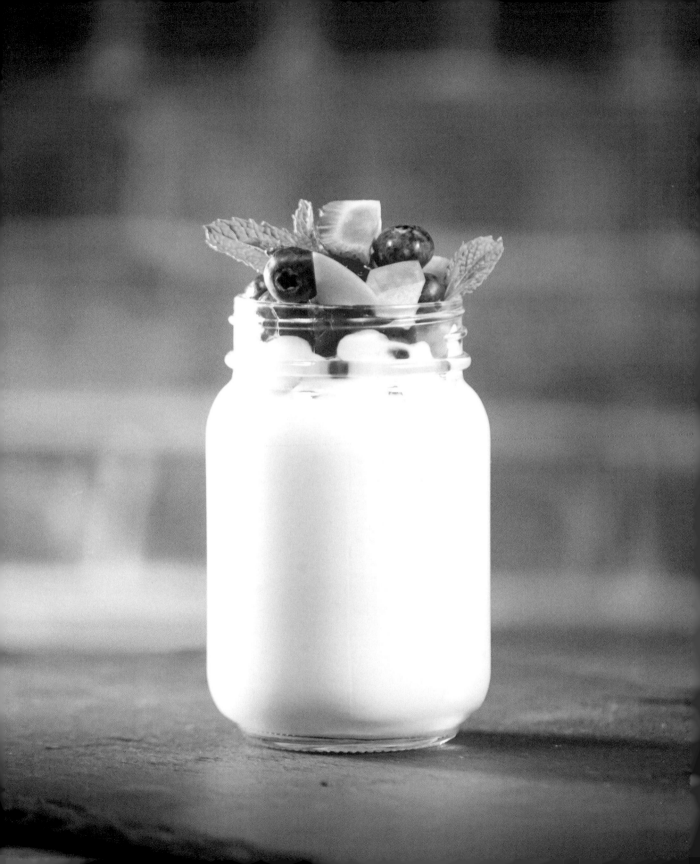

Gut Happy Yogurt

Makes 3 cups

THIS YOGURT MAKES A great addition to smoothies or it can be enjoyed alone. When making yogurt, be sure to use agar-agar *flakes,* not the *powder*. Also, mix things up with different dairy-free milks each week to help diversify your gut microbiome.

¼ cup water

1¾ teaspoons agar-agar flakes

3 cups almond milk *or* coconut milk

1 probiotic capsule with 50 billion CFU

1) Place the water in a small bowl and add the agar-agar flakes. Allow the mixture to rest for about 10 minutes.

2) In a large saucepan over medium-low heat, heat the milk until simmering.

3) Add the water and agar-agar mixture to the saucepan, whisking constantly until the agar-agar has dissolved.

4) Transfer to a bowl and allow it to cool, stirring occasionally, about 15 to 20 minutes, until the mixture registers 110°F on a kitchen thermometer.

5) Twist open the probiotic capsule and whisk the powder into the cooled yogurt mixture; throw away the capsule's casing.

6) Cover the bowl tightly with plastic wrap, place it in your oven, and turn on the oven light. This will add just enough warmth for the culture to grow. Leave the yogurt undisturbed in the oven with the light on for at least 12 hours and up to 24 hours.

7) Chill the yogurt in the refrigerator for at least 4 hours to help it set. To make it creamy smooth, blend it for about 30 seconds in a blender.

8) Store the yogurt in a mason jar with a secure lid in the refrigerator for up to a week.

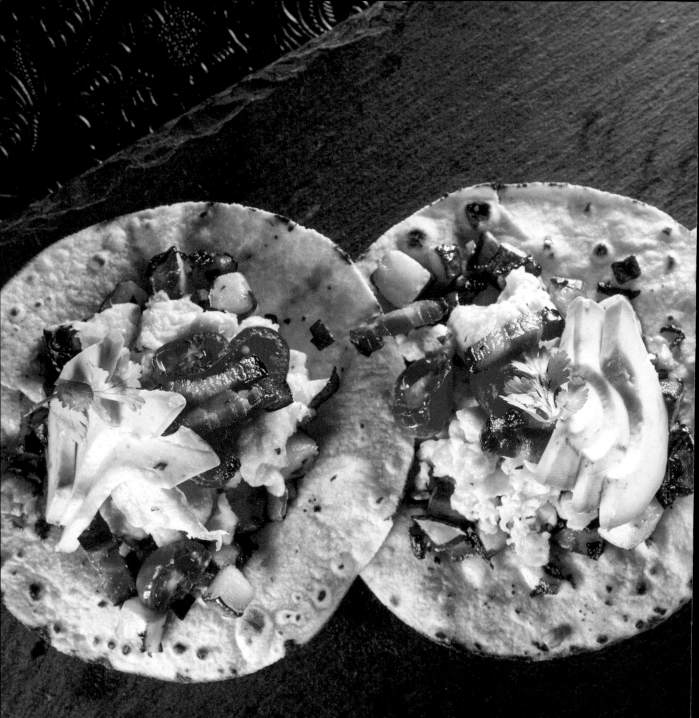

I CAN MAKE A TACO OUT OF ANYTHING. MY HUSBAND LOVES EGG TACOS FOR breakfast, and I prefer bean tacos. I sauté onions and zucchini, and then fold in leftover black beans. Once the veggies are cooked, I stuff them all into a tortilla of choice. For egg lovers, adding homemade mayo to your eggs makes them creamy and delish—I learned this trick in culinary school.

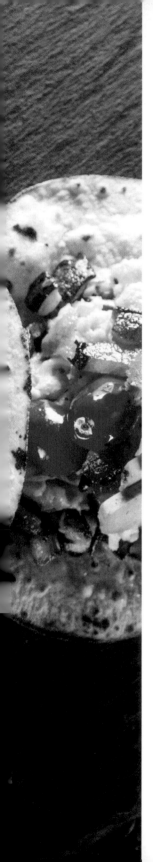

Breakfast Tacos

Makes 4 servings

1 tablespoon extra-virgin olive oil *or* ghee

¼ small onion, diced

1 medium-size zucchini, diced

8 large eggs

1 teaspoon Basic Mayo *(page 212) or* Vegan Mayo *(page 213)*

¼ cup water

½ teaspoon sea salt *(plus more to taste)*

¼ teaspoon black pepper *(plus more to taste)*

6 slices bacon, cooked and crumbled*

8 cornmeal *or* almond flour tortillas *or* Cassava Tortillas** *(page 240)*

½ cup cherry tomatoes, halved

¼ cup thinly sliced scallions

¼ cup chopped cilantro

1 medium avocado, pitted and diced

Substitutions:

*If meat free, replace with Coconut Bacon *(page 157) or* Tempeh Bacon *(page 158)*.

**If grain free, use almond tortillas or Cassava Tortillas. If nut free, use Cassava Tortillas.

1) Heat the oil or ghee in a large skillet over medium heat. Sauté the onions for 3 minutes, and then add the zucchini and cook for 4 minutes, stirring occasionally.

2) In a medium bowl, whisk the eggs with the mayo, water, sea salt, and pepper.

3) Pour the egg mixture into the pan and cook, stirring often, until just set and scrambled, about 3 to 5 minutes. Taste and season with additional sea salt and pepper, if desired. Stir in the bacon crumbles.

4) Warm the tortillas up in a hot skillet. Top each tortilla evenly with eggs, tomatoes, scallions, cilantro, and avocado. Fold it into a taco. Serve immediately.

Cassava Tortillas

Makes 4 servings

YOU CAN'T HAVE
Breakfast Tacos
without the tortilla!
These tortillas are the
gluten-free goodies
that complete a
perfect taco.

1¾ cups plus 1 tablespoon Otto's Naturals Cassava Flour,
plus more for rolling

½ teaspoon sea salt

1 cup hot water

2 tablespoons extra-virgin olive oil

2 tablespoons raw honey *or* maple syrup

1) In a stand mixer fitted with the paddle attachment, combine the flour and sea salt.

2) In a small bowl, whisk together the hot water, oil, and honey or maple syrup. With the mixer running on low, slowly pour the liquid into the flour mixture.

3) Beat on medium speed for about 2 minutes or until the dough is cohesive and not hot to the touch. Divide into 12 balls of equal size. Cover with plastic wrap.

4) Heat a cast-iron skillet over medium heat. While the skillet heats, roll out a ball of dough into a 6-inch tortilla, dusting the dough and your work surface lightly with cassava flour. (You can also roll the dough out between two sheets of parchment paper.)

5) Place the tortilla in the skillet and cook for about 30 seconds. Flip and cook until brown spots appear on the bottom of the tortilla. Transfer to a plate and cover with a clean kitchen towel to keep warm. Repeat the cooking process with the remaining tortillas. (These are best served warm, but they can be made in advance and kept in an airtight container in the refrigerator.)

Dang Good Porridge with Buckwheat and Blueberries

Makes 2 to 4 servings

BUCKWHEAT IS GLUTEN free and, despite its name, it has zero relationship to wheat. It's naturally packed with B vitamins, manganese, copper, magnesium, fiber, and antioxidants. Buckwheat speeds up digestion, which is great if you are constipated or have celiac disease, which can lead to slow mobility. Buckwheat is also pH neutral, making it a great food to eat when you have an upset stomach from too much acid. I love it because it reminds me of cream of wheat. It's soft and easy on my intestines. You can mix this recipe up by rotating your nuts and fruit — figs, bananas, and cooked apples all work great!

3 cups water

1 cup Bob's Red Mill Organic Creamy Buckwheat Hot Cereal

¼ teaspoon sea salt

¼ teaspoon ground cinnamon

1 cup full-fat canned coconut milk *or* other nondairy milk

¼ cup local honey

¼ cup almond butter *or* seed butter

2 cups fresh blueberries

⅓ cup chopped raw walnuts

2 tablespoons chia seeds

1) In a medium pot, bring the water to a boil. Stir in the buckwheat, salt, and cinnamon. Reduce the heat to low and cover. Cook for 8 to 10 minutes, stirring occasionally, until all the water is absorbed.

2) Divide the buckwheat porridge into four serving bowls, and top evenly with the milk, honey, almond butter or seed butter, blueberries, walnuts, and chia seeds. Alternatively, add all the ingredients to the cooked porridge and stir before separating into serving bowls. Enjoy!

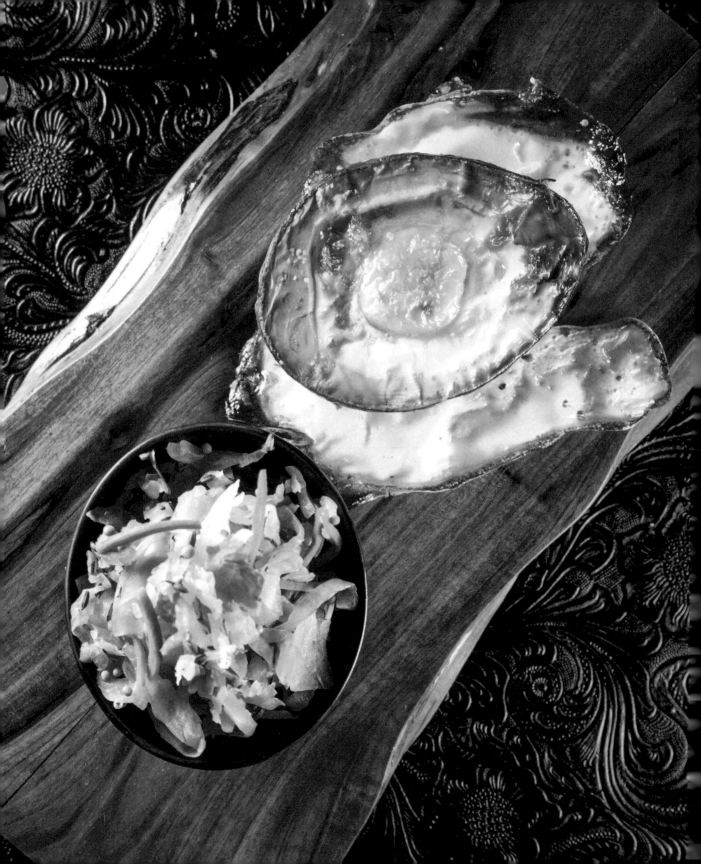

Baked Egg and Avocado with Sauerkraut

Makes 1 serving

THIS IS A MEAL

in itself—it's great for breakfast, brunch, lunch, or dinner. It has a fantastic balance of digestible fat, protein, and probiotics.

1 egg

½ avocado, pit removed and peel intact

1 piece cooked bacon, crumbled*

2 tablespoons fermented probiotic sauerkraut

Freshly ground black pepper *(to taste)*

Sea salt *(to taste)*

Substitutions:

*If meat free, replace with Coconut Bacon *(page 157)* or Tempeh Bacon *(page 158)*.

1) Preheat the oven to 425°F.

2) Remove a little bit of the flesh from the dip in the avocado to make room for the egg if necessary. Slice off a little bit off the bottom of the avocado so that it sits evenly on a baking sheet.

3) Place the avocado on a parchment-lined baking sheet; crack an egg directly into the center of the avocado.

4) Bake for 11 to 15 minutes, depending on how you like your eggs.

5) Top with crumbled bacon and a big old scoop of sauerkraut. Season with pepper and a sprinkle of sea salt. Serve immediately.

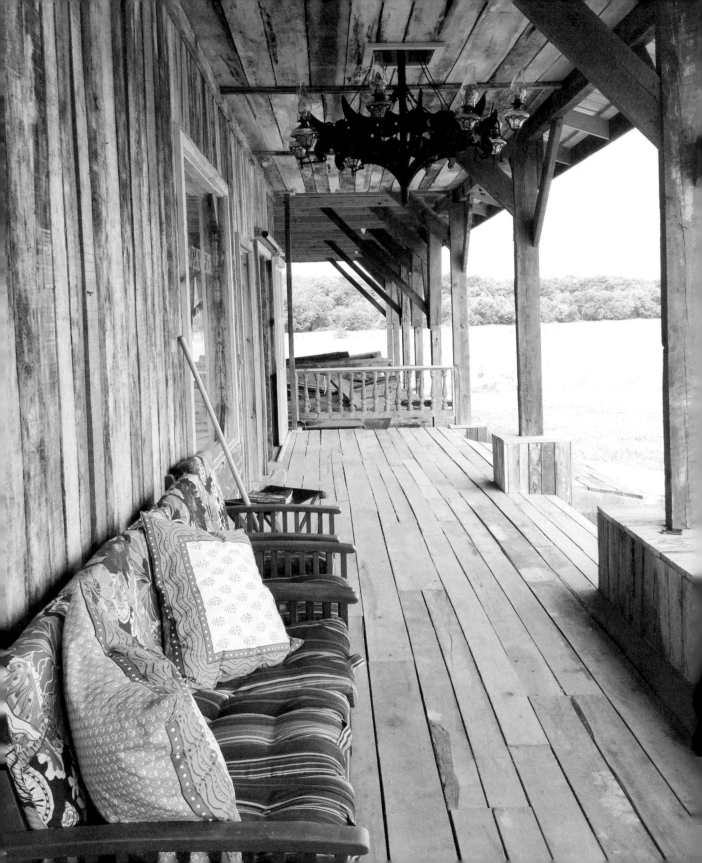

Glorious Gluten-Free Baking & Sweet Endings

I love cakes, biscuits, breads, puddings, and PIE. In fact, I don't know who does not. In Pinewood, we raise the bar each week as we do our best to create new and delicious twists on old classic favorites. The thing to remember with gluten-free baking is that you have to experiment. Each recipe will be slightly different depending upon which gluten-free flour blends you use (see the 411 on different flours on the next page).

Another important tip: Most of these recipes use coconut sugar, which is pretty coarse. For the best results, when baking with coconut sugar, use a spice grinder to grind it to a fine, powdery consistency, which will ensure the perfect texture in your baked goods. It's worth the investment in a good spice grinder.

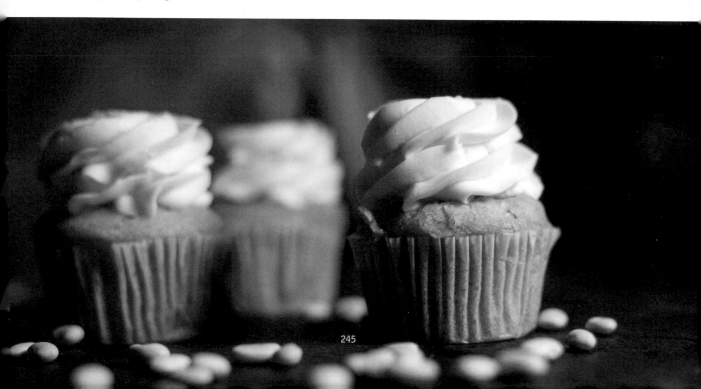

Not All Gluten-Free Flours Are the Same

Here in the United States, the main flour we choose to use for baked goods is wheat, which contains gluten, and it's also the most common allergen. But all over the world, people use flour from different grains and legumes for their baked goods. Here are a few of the flours I like and why:

Amaranth flour. I was first introduced to amaranth while living in Sayulita, Nayarit, in Mexico, as it's very popular there. A benefit of amaranth is that it offers calcium as well as calcium cofactors (minerals that help calcium to be absorbed), and it is high in protein. Amaranth adds a slightly spicy, sweet, and nutty flavor to pancakes, waffles, or muffins, and is usually added in small quantities to leavened products; flatbreads can have more amaranth *(no gluten)*.

Brown rice flour. Brown rice flour has a gentle, nutty taste. It is good in piecrusts or pizza crusts and can be used to make cookies, pancakes, and waffles. Its health benefits include B vitamins and vitamin E *(no gluten)*.

Buckwheat flour. This flour has a very distinct flavor, almost floral. Mixing it with another grain will dilute the floral taste. It contains more protein than many other grains, and it is typically added to pancakes, waffles, and pasta *(no gluten)*.

Cornmeal. Cornmeal is an old-school farm kitchen grain, and it adds a hearty texture to muffins, breads, and polenta. It's the perfect replacer for breadcrumbs as you can coat everything from fish to burgers with it. Blue cornmeal has a higher protein content than yellow cornmeal *(no gluten)*.

Millet flour. This is the least acidic grain, and it's an excellent choice for diabetics. It gives baked goods a subtle taste and works well with other gluten-free flours. For yeast breads, up to 30 percent millet flour may be used. It provides protein, calcium, iron, magnesium, potassium, and phosphorus *(no gluten)*.

Oat flour. Oat flour contains its bran and germ, and is often combined with flours that contain gluten to aid in rising. However, it does not need to be combined with gluten grains; you can balance it with rising agents. It offers a sweet, cake-like crumb that makes it really nice in baked goods. *(It is naturally gluten free but can have gluten if it is processed where gluten grains are also processed.)*

Oat bran. This is a good source of soluble fiber and makes a good substitute for wheat bran. *(It must be marked "gluten free" because it can be cross-contaminated with gluten.)*

Quinoa flour. This flour has a nutty taste. It can be used as the sole flour when making crepes, pancakes, cookies, or muffins. It is a complete protein and contains calcium, iron, phosphorus, vitamin E, and lysine *(no gluten)*.

Tapioca flour. This flour can be used as a thickener, much like traditional wheat flour. It is a great addition to gluten-free breads, giving them a better texture *(no gluten)*.

Mee's Best Bread Ever

Makes 1 loaf

THIS IS AN EASY, QUICK BREAD
that packs a lot of protein, healthy fats, and prebiotic goodness. You can make this totally vegan by replacing the eggs with egg replacer (page 252). Some gluten-free breads are better than others, and this one is the best one I have come across! No yeast, y'all! Now we're talkin'. It's great for French toast, too.

Grapeseed oil spray

2½ cups blanched almond flour

½ teaspoon sea salt

½ teaspoon baking soda

3 large eggs

1 tablespoon honey *or* stevia equivalent *(see page 51)*

½ teaspoon apple cider vinegar

1) Preheat the oven to 300°F. Grease a small loaf pan with grapeseed oil and dust with almond flour.

2) In a large mixing bowl, combine the almond flour, sea salt, and baking soda.

3) In a separate mixing bowl, whisk the eggs, and then add the honey and apple cider vinegar. Fold the wet ingredients into the dry ingredients and blend well.

4) Poor the batter into the greased loaf pan. Bake for 45–55 minutes on the bottom rack of the oven, so the bread doesn't dry out. Cool for at least an hour in the pan. Store in a sealed container in the refrigerator because there are no preservatives.

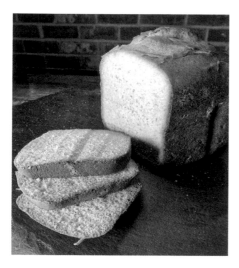

Tip: *When your bread is done, wrap it in a paper towel and store it in a plastic bag in the fridge. Store all homemade breads this way to keep them fresh.*

MASTERING A GLUTEN-FREE BISCUIT THAT ISN'T

a hockey puck is a process, and making it dairy free is another journey altogether. The issue with gluten-free baking is that the protein content is lower, and in this recipe, it is necessary to use psyllium husk because it helps strengthen the protein content — adding an egg helps, too. I also use vegan butter. People light up when we offer them a gluten-free biscuit, and for this, waking up early is worth it. Top one of these with homemade blueberry jam, and it's a good Sunday in Pinewood.

Biscuits

Makes 6 biscuits

1½ cups plus 2 tablespoons King Arthur's Multi-Purpose Flour *or* exactly 9 ounces Bob's Red Mill All-Purpose Flour

4 teaspoons baking powder

1½ teaspoons powdered psyllium husk

1 teaspoon sugar*

½ teaspoon sea salt

¼ teaspoon baking soda

3 tablespoons unsalted vegan butter, chilled, and cut into ¼-inch pieces

¾ cup plain whole-fat coconut milk yogurt *or* goat milk yogurt

1 large egg, lightly beaten

2 tablespoons grapeseed oil

2 teaspoons lemon juice

Substitutions:

*If watching sugar, replace with an equivalent amount of stevia *(page 51)*.

1) In a large bowl, whisk together the flour, baking powder, psyllium husk, sugar, salt, and baking soda until well combined.

2) Add the butter to the flour blend mixture, breaking up the chunks with your fingers until only small, pea-size pieces remain.

3) In a separate bowl, whisk together the yogurt, egg, oil, and lemon juice until well combined.

4) Using a silicone spatula, stir the yogurt mixture into the flour mixture until thoroughly combined and no flour pockets remain, about 1 minute. Cover the bowl with plastic wrap and let the batter rest at room temperature for 30 minutes.

5) Adjust the oven rack to the middle position and preheat the oven to 450°F. Line a rimmed baking sheet with parchment paper. Set the baking sheet atop an additional baking sheet to prevent the bottoms of the biscuits from burning.

6) Using a greased ⅓ cup dry measuring cup, scoop a heaping amount of batter and drop it onto the prepared baking sheet. Space the biscuits about ½ inch apart. Ideally, the biscuits should measure about 2½ inches in diameter and 1½ inches high.

7) Bake until golden and slightly crisp, about 15 minutes, rotating the baking sheet halfway through baking.

8) Transfer the baking sheet to a wire rack and let cool for 5 minutes. These biscuits are best eaten right away.

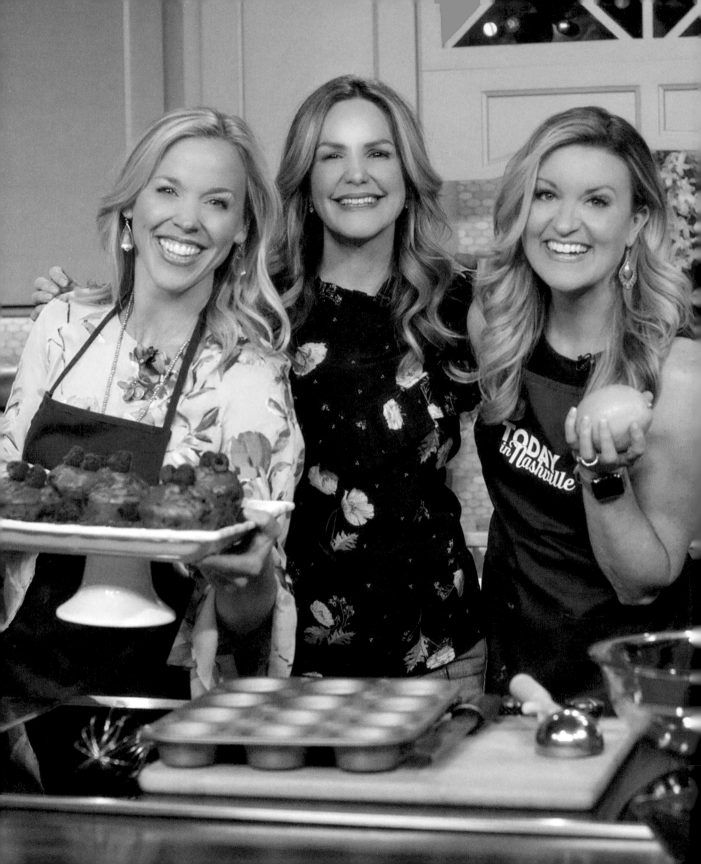

Raspberry Lemonade Muffins

Makes 8 muffins

THESE MUFFINS ARE
grain free and as good as can
be. Dense with protein, they are
lifted up with the lemon and
raspberries for the perfect amount
of brightness. I made them on
Today In Nashville and then we
sold out in Pinewood!

1 cup blanched almond flour *(not almond meal)*

⅛ teaspoon baking soda

⅛ teaspoon sea salt

3 large eggs

¼ cup grapeseed oil

1 tablespoon lemon zest

⅛ teaspoon stevia

1 cup frozen raspberries

1) Preheat the oven to 350°F. In a food processor, pulse the almond flour, baking soda, and salt.

2) Add the eggs, grapeseed oil, lemon zest, and stevia and pulse for about 20 seconds.

3) Remove the blade and fold in the raspberries by hand. Divide the batter between 8 muffin cups and bake for 30 minutes.

Egg Replacers

For the first year on my new healing-with-food journey, I avoided eggs completely. Every time I'd eat anything containing eggs, I'd get a tingling sensation in my mouth and a nauseous tummy. I was all about avoiding them, and now that I cook and bake for folks with food allergies, I've mastered the egg replacer!

Speedy Egg Replacer with Flax Meal

Equal to 1 egg

1 tablespoon ground flax meal

2½ tablespoons water

Mix the ingredients together and allow to rest for 5 minutes before using in a recipe as an egg substitute.

Speedy Egg Replacer with Psyllium Seed Husks

Equal to 1 egg

PSYLLIUM SEED HUSKS are soluble fiber. Psyllium helps relieve diarrhea, constipation, and irritable bowel syndrome (IBS). It helps maintain and improve GI transit. It also helps lower cholesterol and controls diabetes. This egg replacer can be used in gluten-free baking and helps make the bread crumble less.

1 tablespoon psyllium seed husks

2 tablespoons water

Mix the ingredients together and allow to rest for 5 minutes before using in a recipe as an egg substitute.

Here are some more easy alternatives for eggs; all are equivalent to 1 egg in a recipe:

- For desserts or smoothies, use ½ medium or large banana.
- For sweeter recipes, use 3 tablespoons to ¼ cup applesauce.
- Blend ¼ cup soft or silken tofu in a food processor.
- Buy an egg replacer product found in most health food stores, and use 1½ teaspoons with 2 tablespoons water.

Dinner Rolls

HAVING CELIAC DISEASE MEANS I ALWAYS HAVE TO PASS ON THE DINNER ROLLS
when eating out — but not in Pinewood. These babies are a treat and something I make at home on special occasions.

1⅓ cups warm water *(110°F)* plus 1 teaspoon water

2 teaspoons lemon juice

2 large eggs plus 1 large yolk

3½ cups 1-to-1 gluten-free flour blend

½ cup nonfat nondairy milk powder, organic milk powder, *or* goat's milk powder

2 tablespoons powdered psyllium husk

2 tablespoons finely ground coconut sugar

2¼ teaspoons instant *or* rapid-rise yeast

2 teaspoons baking powder

½ teaspoon sea salt plus a pinch

6 tablespoons unsalted vegan *or* grass-fed butter, cut into 6 pieces and softened

Substitutions:

*If watching sugar, use an equivalent amount of stevia *(page 51)*.

1) Spray a 9-inch round cake pan with grapeseed oil spray.

2) In a bowl, whisk together the warm water, lemon juice, 1 of the eggs, and the yolk. Set aside.

3) Using a stand mixer fitted with a paddle, on low speed, mix together the flour, milk powder, psyllium husk, sugar, yeast, baking powder, and sea salt until combined. Slowly add the water mixture and let the dough come together, about 1 minute, scraping down the bowl as needed.

4) Add the butter, increase the speed to medium, and beat until sticky and uniform, about 6 minutes.

5) Working with one-third cup of the dough at a time, shape into rough rounds using wet hands. Arrange the rolls in the prepared pan (one in the center and seven spaced evenly around the edges). Cover loosely with plastic wrap and let rise at room temperature until the dough doubles in size (the rolls should press against each other), about 1 hour. (Risen rolls can be refrigerated for up to 4 hours.)

6) Adjust the oven rack to the middle position and preheat the oven to 375°F. In a bowl, lightly beat the remaining egg with 1 teaspoon of water and the pinch of salt until combined.

7) Remove the plastic and brush the rolls with the egg wash. Bake until the tops are golden brown, 35 to 40 minutes, rotating the pan halfway through baking.

8) Let the rolls cool in the pan on a wire rack for 10 minutes, then invert onto a rack; reinvert rolls and let them cool for 10 to 15 minutes. Break the rolls apart and serve warm.

I AM OBSESSED WITH OLD SOUTHERN COOKBOOKS—I MEAN OLD LIKE FROM the 1800s. I am always sorting through recipes and sending them to my sister, Nicole. She makes old-school skillet cornbread. I love the crispiness and the soft warm center that results when it's made in a skillet. This is comfort food number-one in my mind. These steps might feel like a lot of work, but they're necessary for adding layers of flavor and creating the crisp crust and moist center.

Skillet Cornbread

Makes 8 to 10 servings

2¼ cups cornmeal*

1½ cups Cashew Sour Cream *(page 213)*
   or store-bought dairy
   or nondairy sour cream

½ cup oat milk

¼ cup grapeseed oil

4 tablespoons unsalted grass-fed butter
   or vegan butter

2 tablespoons light brown sugar *or*
   finely ground coconut sugar**

1 teaspoon baking powder

1 teaspoon baking soda

¾ teaspoon sea salt

2 large eggs

Optional:

diced red pepper

diced jalapeños

Substitutions:

*If corn free, use almond meal.

**If watching sugar, use an equivalent amount of stevia *(page 51)*.

1) Adjust the oven racks to the lower-middle and middle positions and preheat the oven to 450°F. Place a 10-inch cast-iron skillet on the middle rack and heat for 10 minutes.

2) Meanwhile, spread the cornmeal over a rimmed baking sheet and toast in the oven on the lower-middle rack until fragrant and lightly golden, about 5 minutes.

3) Carefully transfer the toasted cornmeal to a large bowl and whisk in the sour cream and milk; set aside. When the skillet is hot, add the oil and continue to heat until just smoking, about 5 minutes.

4) Using potholders (the skillet handle will be hot), remove the skillet from the oven, carefully add the butter, and gently swirl to incorporate. Pour the hot oil-butter mixture into the cornmeal mixture and whisk to incorporate. Whisk in the sugar, baking powder, baking soda, and salt, followed by the eggs. If you want to add some heat or texture, fold in the optional jalepeños or red pepper.

5) Quickly scrape the batter into a hot skillet and smooth out the top. Bake on the middle rack until it begins to crackle and appears golden brown, about 12 to 15 minutes, rotating the skillet halfway through baking.

Pignoli

Makes about 12 cookies

THESE ARE MY GREAT grandmother's cookies. They are also my grandma's favorite cookie. They remind me so much of home that I bake them just to smell them.

1⅔ cups slivered blanched almonds *or* 14 ounces
  gluten-free marzipan

1⅓ cups light brown sugar *or* finely ground coconut sugar*

2 large egg whites

1 cup pine nuts

Substitutions:

*If watching sugar, use an equivalent amount of stevia
(page 51).

1) Adjust the oven racks to the upper-middle and lower-middle positions and preheat the oven to 350°F. Line two baking sheets with parchment paper.

2) In a food processor, process the almonds and sugar until finely ground, about 30 seconds. Scrape down the sides and add the egg whites. Continue to process until smooth (the dough will be wet), about 30 seconds; transfer the mixture to a bowl. Place the pine nuts in a shallow dish.

3) Working with 1 scant tablespoon of dough at a time, roll into balls, roll in the pine nuts to coat, and space 2 inches apart on the prepared baking sheets.

4) Bake the cookies until light golden brown, for 13 to 15 minutes, switching and rotating the baking sheets halfway through baking.

5) Let the cookies cool on sheets for 5 minutes, and then transfer to a wire rack. Cool the cookies to room temperature before serving.

Piecrust

Makes 1 pie crust

3 tablespoons ice water

1½ tablespoons Cashew Sour Cream *(page 213) or* Coconut Sour Cream *(page 214)*

1½ teaspoons rice vinegar

¾ cup plus ⅔ cup 1-to-1 gluten-free flour blend*

1½ teaspoons finely ground coconut sugar**

½ teaspoon sea salt

¼ teaspoon ground psyllium husk *or* ground flax

¼-inch piece organic all-vegetable shortening

Substitutions:

*If grain free, use almond flour.

**If watching sugar, use an equivalent amount of stevia *(page 51).*

1) In a medium bowl, stir together the ice water, sour cream, and vinegar.

2) In a food processor, combine the flour, sugar, salt, and ground psyllium or flax, and process for about 5 seconds. Scatter the shortening over the top and pulse until the crumbs look uniform and the shortening is no longer visible, about 20 to 30 pulses.

3) Pour the sour cream mixture over the flour mixture and pulse until the dough comes together in large pieces, about 20 pulses.

4) Lay down a piece of plastic wrap, and then on top of it, lay down a piece of parchment paper. Turn the dough out onto the parchment paper and flatten into a 5-inch disk. Wrap the parchment and plastic around the dough and refrigerate for an hour. (This keeps the plastic from touching the dough.)

5) Allow the dough to sit on the counter for about 20 minutes to soften. Roll the dough into a 12-inch circle between two large sheets of parchment paper, and then gently peel apart and invert the dough over a 9-inch pie plate. Ease the dough in gently. Tuck any overhanging dough under itself to be flush with the edge of the pie plate. Crimp the dough evenly around the edge using your fingers. Cover the dough loosely and put it in the freezer just until chilled, about 15 minutes.

6) Adjust the oven rack to the lower-middle position and preheat the oven to 375°F. Bake the crust until crisp and golden, about 25 minutes. Remove the pie crust from the oven and fill it with whatever makes you happiest.

Substitutions:

*If watching sugar, use an equivalent amount of stevia *(page 51)*.

Substitutions:

**If watching sugar, use an equivalent amount of stevia *(page 51)*; however, coconut nectar is low glycemic.

Vegan Chocolate Fudge Brownies with Homemade Strawberry Jam

Makes 4 servings

FOR THE BROWNIES:

4 tablespoons ground chia seeds

½ cup plus 2 tablespoons water

⅔ cup coconut oil

1¾ cups finely ground coconut sugar*

1 teaspoon pure vanilla extract

1 cup cocoa powder

1 cup plus 2 tablespoons coconut flour

¾ teaspoon baking powder

¾ teaspoon fine sea salt

¾ cup vegan semisweet dark chocolate, chopped into chunks

FOR THE JAM:

1 pound fresh strawberries, roughly chopped

¼ cup local honey *or* coconut nectar**

2 tablespoons chia seeds

½ teaspoon pure vanilla extract

Pinch fine sea salt

TO MAKE THE BROWNIES:

1) Combine the ground chia seeds and water in a bowl. Whisk to combine. Wait at least 10 minutes for the consistency to become egg-like.

2) In a saucepan over medium heat, melt the coconut oil; add the coconut sugar and the vanilla extract. Stir to combine until it's liquid in texture.

3) Sift the cocoa powder and coconut flour into a large mixing bowl; add the baking powder and sea salt, and mix to combine. Combine the chia seed mixture and the melted coconut oil/sugar mixture. Stir to combine, but don't overmix. Add the chocolate and stir again to combine.

4) Preheat the oven to 350°F. Line a 7-x-7-inch baking dish with parchment paper and pour the brownie mix into the dish; smooth with a spatula. Bake for 30 minutes or until a toothpick inserted comes out clean. Let cool before cutting. Serve topped with spoonfuls of jam.

TO MAKE THE JAM:

1) In a saucepan on medium-high heat, cook the strawberries, stirring often, until they begin to soften and release their water. Reduce the heat to low.

2) Add the honey or nectar, chia seeds, vanilla extract, and sea salt, and simmer, stirring occasionally, until the liquid is reduced by half. Remove from the heat and let sit for at least 15 minutes to thicken. If desired, add more honey or nectar, to taste.

FOR THE ICING:

1 cup raw cashews, soaked overnight and strained *or* roasted salt-free cashews*

¼ cup full-fat coconut milk

1 teaspoon pure vanilla extract

2 teaspoons local honey

1 teaspoon lemon juice

1 teaspoon apple cider vinegar

Pinch fine sea salt

4 to 6 tablespoons unsweetened almond milk *or* oat milk *or* coconut milk

¼ cup walnuts, chopped *(optional for topping)*

Decorative sprinkles *(optional)*

Substitutions:

*If nut free, replace with vegan butter that's not made from nuts, such as Earth Balance.

Substitutions:

**If watching sugar, replace with an equivalent amount of stevia *(page 51).*

Vegan Carrot Cake with Vanilla Cashew Icing

Makes 4 to 6 servings

FOR THE CAKE:

⅓ cup melted coconut oil, plus more for the pan

1½ cups 1-to-1 gluten-free flour blend, plus more for dusting the pan

3 tablespoons ground chia seeds

½ cup plus 1 tablespoon water

¼ cup agave nectar

¾ cup unsweetened applesauce

¾ cup finely ground coconut sugar**

1 teaspoon fine sea salt

1½ teaspoons baking soda

1½ teaspoons baking powder

1½ teaspoons ground cinnamon

1 teaspoon ground ginger

¾ cup unsweetened almond milk *or* oat milk

1½ cups grated carrots, tightly packed

1½ cups blanched almond flour

¾ cups chopped walnuts

¼ cup organic raisins

¼ cup dried pineapple *(optional)*

1) Lightly grease a 9-inch Bundt pan with coconut oil and dust with flour. Shake out the excess flour and set aside.

2) In a bowl, whisk together the ground chia seeds and water. Wait at least 10 minutes until they form an egg-like consistency. Set aside and preheat the oven to 350°F.

3) In a large mixing bowl, combine the coconut oil, agave nectar, applesauce, sugar, sea salt, baking soda, baking powder, cinnamon, ginger, milk, and the chia mixture. Whisk to combine. Add the grated carrot and flours and mix to combine. (The batter should have a normal batter consistency; if it's too thick, add milk a little at a time.) Stir in the chopped walnuts, raisins, and dried pineapple (if using).

4) Pour the batter into the Bundt pan, and bake for 40 to 45 minutes, or until a toothpick inserted comes out clean. Remove from the oven and let it cool for at least 15 minutes before flipping the pan to remove the cake.

5) While the cake cools, make the icing. In a blender, combine the soaked and strained cashews, coconut milk, vanilla extract, honey, lemon juice, vinegar, and sea salt. Blend or pulse to combine. While blending, slowly pour in 4 to 6 tablespoons of milk until the icing blends into a smooth, creamy, and pourable mixture.

6) Gently pour the icing over the cake, using enough to coat the cake as desired. Top with chopped walnuts and decorative sprinkles (if using). Slice the cake and serve with the remaining icing.

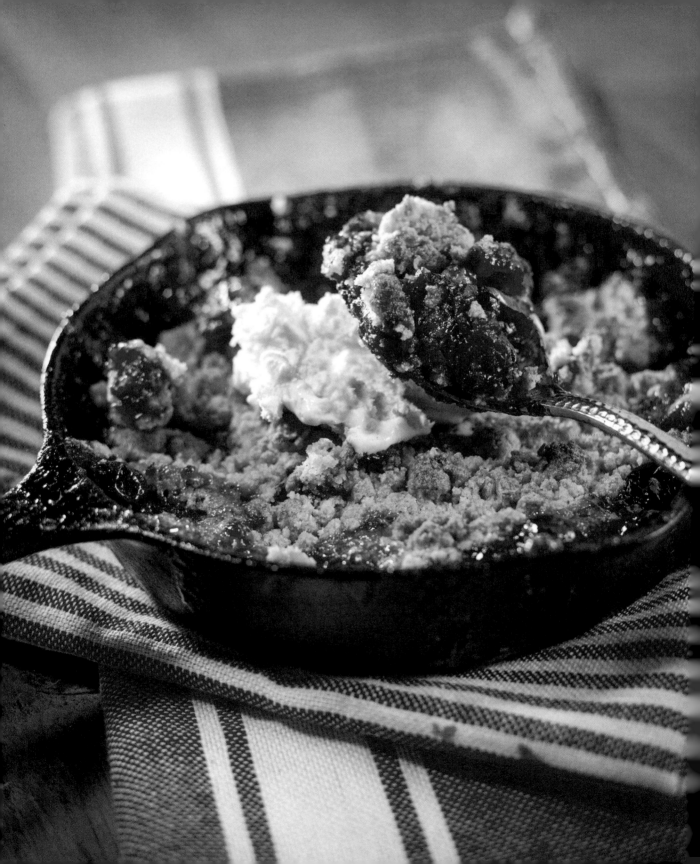

Tangy Cranberry Cobbler

Makes 4 to 6 servings

I LOVE THIS FOR

a holiday dessert. Starting in November, grocery stores sell fresh cranberries, and I go cranberry crazy.

2 cups thawed frozen *or* fresh cranberries

1 cup dried cranberries

1 cup raisins

½ cup orange juice

¼ cup plus 2 tablespoons finely ground coconut sugar*, divided

2 teaspoons arrowroot powder *or* kuzu root

1 cup 1-to-1 gluten-free flour blend**

2 teaspoons baking powder

1 teaspoon ground cinnamon

¼ teaspoon sea salt

¼ cup grass-fed butter *or* organic all-vegetable shortening, cut into small pieces

½ cup nondairy milk

Substitutions:

*If watching sugar, use an equivalent amount of stevia *(page 51)*.

**If grain free, use 1½ cups almond flour.

1) Preheat the oven to 400°F. Combine the cranberries, dried cranberries, raisins, orange juice, ¼ cup of the sugar, and arrowroot powder or kuzu root in a 9-inch square baking dish; toss to coat.

2) Combine the flour, the remaining 2 tablespoons of coconut sugar, baking powder, cinnamon, and sea salt in large bowl; mix well. Cut in the butter or shortening until the mixture resembles coarse crumbs. Add the milk; stir until just moistened.

3) Drop the batter by large spoonfuls over the cranberry mixture. Bake for 35 to 40 minutes or until the topping is golden brown. Serve warm.

I AM SO VERY PROUD of these fry pies. Maybe it's because Pinewood Kitchen's Ms. Tina had never heard the words "vegan" or "gluten free" before working with us or maybe it's because gluten-free and vegan folks hadn't had pie — let alone a fry pie — in years and they light up when they taste them! We stuff these babies with whatever fruit or berries we've got. Apples are a good place to start.

Substitutions:
*If grain free, use almond flour.

Ms. Tina's Pinewood Apple Fry Pies

Makes 8 servings

FOR THE APPLE FILLING:

2 tablespoons coconut oil

4 pounds apples, peeled, cored, and chopped

1½ teaspoons cinnamon

¼ teaspoon nutmeg

1½ cups finely ground coconut sugar

3 tablespoons arrowroot powder

3 tablespoons water

FOR THE DOUGH:

8 cups 1-to-1 gluten-free flour blend*

2 teaspoons baking powder

1 cup finely ground coconut sugar

2 teaspoons baking soda

1 cup crumbled organic all-vegetable shortening

5 to 6 cups ice water

1 cup grapeseed oil for frying

TO MAKE THE APPLE FILLING:

1) In a large skillet over medium heat, melt the oil. Add the apples, cinnamon, nutmeg, and sugar. Cover and cook, stirring occasionally, for 4 to 6 minutes or until the apples are very slightly softened.

2) In a small bowl, combine the arrowroot powder and water. While stirring the apples, drizzle in the diluted arrowroot powder and continue to cook until the apples are soft and the filling is thickened. Let bubble for 1 minute. Remove from the heat and cool completely.

TO MAKE THE DOUGH AND FRY PIES:

1) In a large bowl, whisk together the flour, baking powder, and baking soda. Add the shortening and mix thoroughly until the mixture forms pea-size, messy (aka "shaggy") crumbles. Add the ice water to the mixture until it forms a soft dough that holds together.

2) Roll the dough out onto a surface dusted with gluten-free flour. Using a rolling pin, flatten to an ⅛ to ¼-inch thickness. Using a 6-inch bowl as a guide, cut into circles.

3) Add 4 to 5 tablespoons of apple filling onto one half of the pie. Fold over the top of the dough and crimp the edges to seal in the fruit.

4) Heat the oil in a deep Dutch oven until it reaches 350°F. Drop in the fry pies and cook for 3 to 4 minutes. Remove the fry pies from the pan with a slotted spoon and drain on paper towels.

I MAKE PIES OUT OF ALL KINDS OF PUMPKINS.
My favorite is the North Georgia Candy Roaster.
It's a 500-year-old Cherokee Indian heirloom
seed that we continue to grow in Pinewood.
It's long and oddly shaped, but the flesh is
orange and rich. When it arrives on the farm,
we all do the happy dance because we know
how good the pies are going to be.

Pumpkin Pie

Makes 8 servings

1 Piecrust *(page 257)*

1 *(15-ounce)* can pumpkin puree *or* 2 cups freshly cooked pumpkin puree

1½ cups finely ground coconut sugar*

2 teaspoons ground ginger

2 teaspoons ground cinnamon

1 teaspoon ground nutmeg

½ teaspoon sea salt

¼ teaspoon ground cloves

⅔ cup whole-fat coconut cream

⅔ cup nondairy milk

4 large eggs

Substitutions:

*If watching sugar, use an equivalent amount of stevia *(page 51)*.

1) Adjust the oven rack to the middle position and heat the oven to 375°F. Bake the piecrust until light brown in color, about 20 to 25 minutes, rotating the pie plate halfway through baking. Transfer the pie plate to a wire rack. (The crust must still be warm when the filling is added.) Adjust the oven rack to the lower position and increase the oven temperature to 425°F.

2) While the crust bakes, in a food processor, process the pumpkin, sugar, ginger, cinnamon, nutmeg, sea salt, and cloves until combined, about 1 minute.

3) Transfer the pumpkin mixture to a medium saucepan (do not clean the processor bowl) and bring to a simmer over medium-high heat. Cook the pumpkin mixture, stirring constantly, until it's thick and shiny, about 5 minutes. Whisk in the cream and nondairy milk, return to simmer briefly, and then remove from the heat.

4) Whip the eggs in the food processor until uniform, about 5 seconds. With the machine running, slowly add about half of the hot pumpkin mixture through the feed tube. Stop the machine, add the remaining pumpkin, and continue processing the mixture until it's uniform in texture, about 30 seconds longer.

5) Immediately pour the warm filling into the partially baked piecrust. (If you have any extra filling, ladle it into the pie after 5 minutes of baking, by which time the filling will have settled.) Bake until the filling is puffed and lightly cracked around the edges and the center wiggles slightly when jiggled, about 25 minutes. Let the pie cool on a wire rack until the filling has set, about 2 hours; serve slightly warm or at room temperature.

Five-Ingredient Fudge Cups

Makes 4 servings

PURE COCOA POWDER IS packed with antioxidants that help protect our cells. Since 1 tablespoon contains 12.42 mg of caffeine, if you're looking for a little caffeine pick-me-up midafternoon, this little treat is perfect. If you want to skip the caffeine, swap out the dark chocolate for carob chips.

1 cup vegan dark chocolate chips *or* carob chips

6 tablespoons full-fat coconut milk

1 tablespoon coconut oil

1 teaspoon pure vanilla extract

Pinch sea salt

1) Using a mini muffin tin, line 12 mini muffin cups with paper liners.

2) In a double boiler set over gently simmering water, combine the chips, coconut milk, and coconut oil. Stir often until melted. Remove from the heat and stir in the vanilla extract and sea salt.

3) Divide among the prepared muffin cups. Refrigerate for 1 hour or freeze for 30 minutes, until set.

Feed Your Gut Some Carob

Carob comes from the pod of a bush that grows along the Mediterranean Sea. Inside the pod is a sweet pulp. It's dried and roasted, then ground into a powder called carob powder. This powder is then formed into chips. It's similar to cocoa powder and can be substituted 1 to 1 in recipes. Carob's health benefits are many. It's high in protein since it comes from the legume family, and contains vitamins A, B, B3, and D. What really stands out is that it's an excellent source of calcium.

Why do gut bacteria like it? Because it's a prebiotic food and a digestive aid, and traditionally, it was used to soothe an upset stomach. We now know that upset tummies mean an upset in the gut bacteria community. Feed the healthy bacteria and you bring the gut back into balance. For a cold winter night treat, try making hot carob and coconut milk instead of hot cocoa.

Individual Chocolate Soufflés

Makes 2 servings

CHOCOLATE anything is amazing —but *warm* chocolate is what I want when it comes to dessert. This recipe brings delicious cacao and all its prebiotic goodness to the table or your mug.

1 tablespoon vegan butter *or* grass-fed butter, plus more for greasing

2 tablespoons plus 1 teaspoon finely ground coconut sugar*, divided

4 ounces bittersweet dark vegan chocolate, broken into pieces, *or* carob chips

2 eggs, separated, at room temperature

A dusting of powdered sugar *(optional)*

Substitutions:

*If watching sugar, use an equivalent amount of stevia *(page 51)*.

1) Preheat the oven to 375°F. Coat two (6-ounce) soufflé dishes or ramekins with butter. Add ½ teaspoon coconut sugar to each dish; shake to coat bottoms and sides.

2) Combine the chocolate or carob and 1 tablespoon of the butter in the top of a double boiler; heat over simmering water until the chocolate or carob is melted and smooth, stirring occasionally. Remove from the heat; stir in the egg yolks, one at a time, until blended. The mixture may become grainy but will smooth out with the addition of the egg whites.

3) Beat the egg whites in a medium bowl with an electric mixer at high speed until soft peaks form. Gradually add the remaining 2 tablespoons of sugar; beat until stiff peaks form and the mixture is glossy.

4) Gently fold the egg whites into the chocolate or carob mixture. Do not overmix; allow some white streaks to remain. Divide the batter evenly between prepared dishes.

5) Bake for 15 minutes until the soufflés rise but are moist in the centers. Dust with the powdered sugar, if desired. Serve immediately.

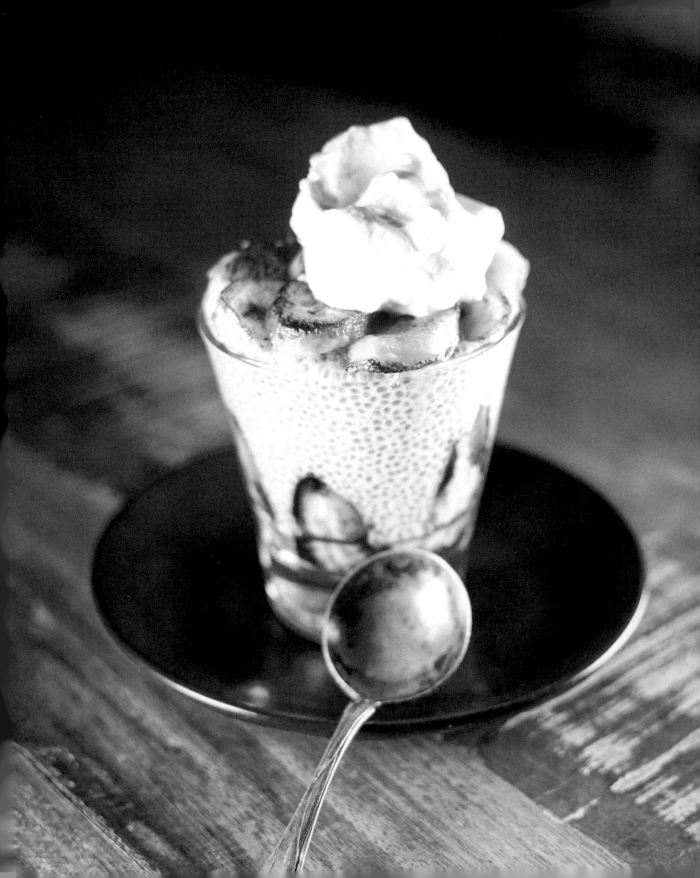

Vegan Banana Cream Chia Seed Pudding

Makes 2 servings

THIS RECIPE SHOULD be renamed The Dessert No One Can Mess Up because it is the simplest recipe ever. It tastes great and is super healthy with the omega-rich oils from the chia seeds and the potassium from the banana. I like to garnish with some fresh blueberries because blueberries make everything better.

FOR THE PUDDING BASE:

3 tablespoons chia seeds

1 cup dairy-free milk

1 large banana *(ripe but firm)*, peeled and halved

FOR THE TOPPING:

½ tablespoon coconut oil

1 banana, peeled and sliced into rounds

1) In a jar, mix together the chia seeds and milk. Cover and refrigerate for at least 2 hours or overnight.

2) Mash the banana and stir it into the chia seed pudding. Stir in more milk if a thinner consistency is desired.

3) Heat up the oil in a cast-iron pan over medium-high heat. Add the banana slices. Cook for about a minute before flipping with a fork; they will release from the pan when they are done. Add the warm bananas to the top of the chia pudding, and enjoy. You can also make a parfait instead. Just layer half of the cooked bananas on the bottom of a glass jar and then layer with the pudding and then top with the rest of the cooked bananas.

Grain-Free Lava Cake

Makes 6 servings

YUMMY, EASY, AND LOADED WITH ANTIOXIDANT COCOA, THIS CAKE IS MY JAM.
If you serve it with some fresh raspberries or sliced strawberries on top and a scoop of ice cream on the side, you will be in heaven.

Grapeseed oil cooking spray

2 to 3 tablespoons cocoa powder, plus more for dusting cakes

5 ounces dark chocolate *(at least 71% cacao)*

10 tablespoons unsalted grass-fed butter *or* vegan butter

1 cup finely ground coconut sugar*

3 tablespoons arrowroot powder

3 large eggs, separated

2 tablespoons coconut flour

Substitutions:

*If watching sugar, use an equivalent amount of stevia *(page 51)*.

1) Spray six (6-ounce) ramekins with grapeseed oil cooking spray and dust with the cocoa powder.

2) Combine the chocolate and butter in a large glass bowl and set over a pot of simmering water on the stovetop. Melt and whisk until smooth.

3) Remove the chocolate mixture from the heat and let it cool for 5 minutes.

4) Add the finely ground coconut sugar, arrowroot powder, egg yolks, and coconut flour to the chocolate mixture and whisk until smooth. Whisk the egg whites until they are slightly fluffy and fold them into the batter. Spoon the batter evenly into ramekins.

5) Freeze for at least 5 hours or overnight.

6) Adjust the oven rack to the middle position, and preheat the oven to 450°F. Line a baking sheet with parchment paper.

7) Transfer the frozen cakes to the prepared baking sheet, and bake for 18 minutes.

8) Remove the cakes from the oven and let them cool for no longer than 3 minutes so that they can be served hot.

9) Using a kitchen knife, cut around the edge of the cakes and gently lift each cake onto a serving dish. Top with Whipped Coconut Cream (page 280) and a dusting of cocoa powder. Serve immediately.

Key Lime Avocado Tart

Makes 4 servings

I MADE THIS

recipe on *The Better Show,* and so many people wrote to me about it that I couldn't keep up. I like to serve this in the summer, and it makes me so happy when my avocado "dislikers" LOVE it. You can make this ahead, keep it in the freezer, and pull it out when you're ready to serve up an elegant dessert.

FOR THE CRUST:

¼ cup unsweetened shredded coconut

½ cup chopped pecans

10 pitted dates *(about ½ cup)*

2 teaspoons lime zest

Pinch sea salt

Grapeseed oil cooking spray

FOR THE FILLING:

2 avocados, peeled and pitted

½ cup freshly squeezed lime juice

¼ cup local honey

1 heaping tablespoon coconut oil

2 teaspoons lime zest

3 tablespoons coconut milk

TO MAKE THE CRUST:

1) In a food processor, combine the coconut, pecans, dates, lime zest, and sea salt, and process until well combined and a sticky paste forms.

2) Press the paste evenly into three mini springform pans with removable bottoms coated with grapeseed oil spray.

TO MAKE THE FILLING AND ASSEMBLE THE TART:

1) In a clean food processor, combine all the filling ingredients and puree until very smooth.

2) Pour the tart filling over your crusts, smoothing out the tops so they freeze evenly. Cover and place in the freezer for 2 hours. Allow to thaw for 10 minutes before serving.

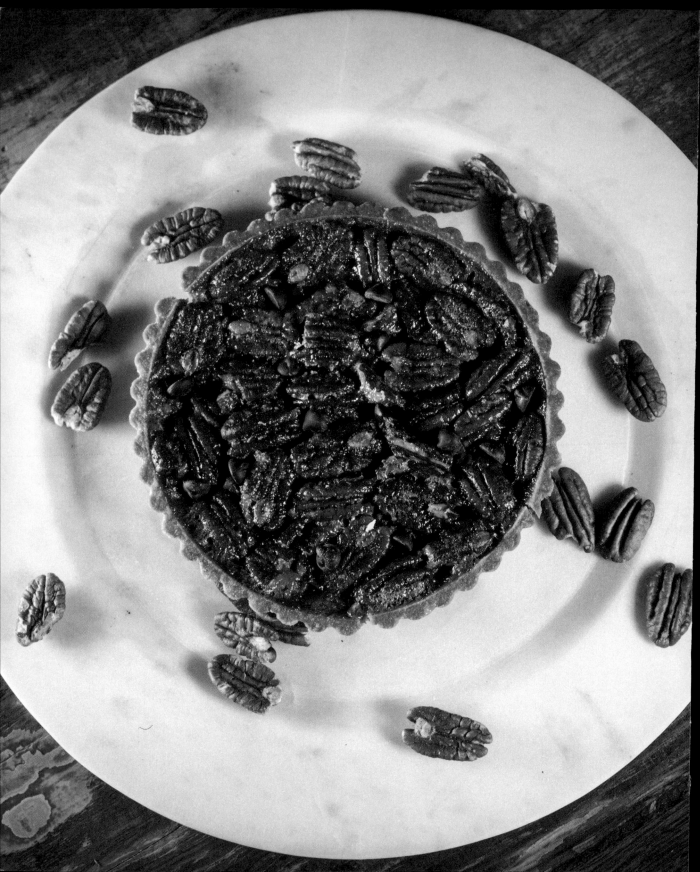

Healthier Holiday Pecan–Coconut Carob Chip Pie with Almond Meal Crust

Makes 8 servings or 4 individual mini pies

FOR THE PIE CRUST:

3 cups blanched almond meal flour *or* cashew meal flour

¼ teaspoon sea salt

½ cup finely ground coconut sugar *(optional)*

1 teaspoon cinnamon

3 tablespoons coconut oil

1 egg

FOR THE FILLING:

4 large eggs

1 cup finely ground coconut sugar

1 cup coconut nectar

½ cup coconut oil, melted

1 tablespoon coconut milk

2 cups chopped pecans

1 cup carob chips *or* dairy-free chocolate chips

Substitution:

*If watching sugar, replace with an equivalent amount of stevia *(page 51)*.

TO MAKE THE PIECRUST:

1) In a food processor, combine the almond meal or cashew meal flour, sea salt, coconut sugar, and cinnamon, and pulse briefly. Add the coconut oil and egg, pulsing until the mixture forms a ball.

2) Press the dough into a 9-inch pie pan or into four mini pie tins. Do not prebake the crust. Preheat the oven to 350°F.

TO MAKE THE FILLING AND ASSEMBLE THE PIE:

1) In a food processor or blender, combine the eggs, coconut sugar, coconut nectar, melted coconut oil, and coconut milk, and blend until completely uniform. Remove the blade, add the pecans and chips, and fold them in by hand.

2) Pour the filling into the piecrust. Bake the pie for 40 to 50 minutes, until the middle is firm. If making mini pies, check after 30 minutes to avoid drying them out. Serve with a dollop of Whipped Coconut Cream (page 280).

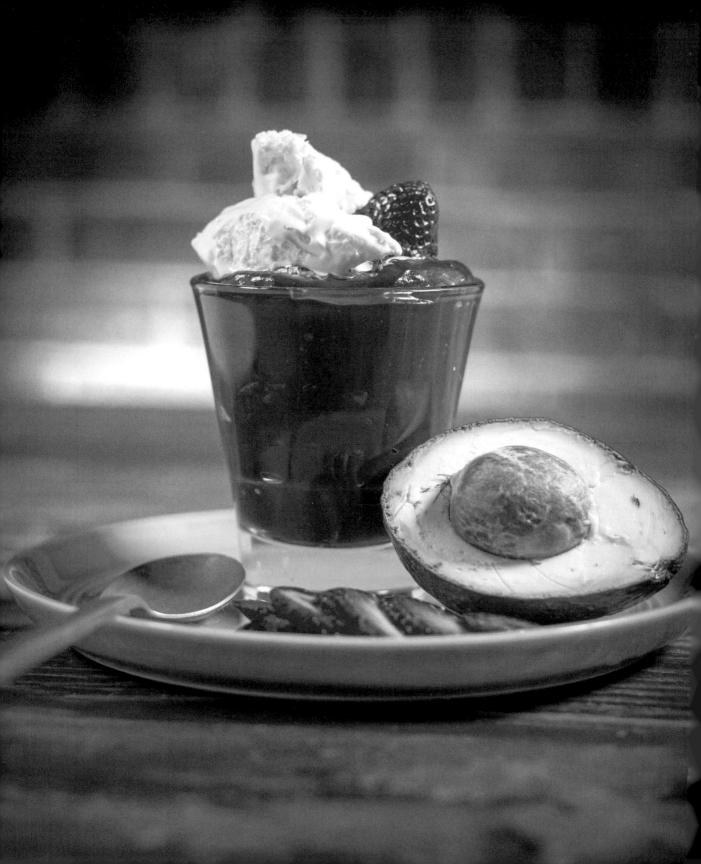

Chocolate—Avocado Mousse

Makes 4 servings

EVERYONE I KNOW LOVES this mousse—and no one can tell that this one is made with avocados. If you can taste the avocado, add more cacao next time. It's a great way to use up older avocados that are starting to brown a little. Garnish with fresh fruit or chopped nuts.

I like to serve this mousse with whipped coconut cream—YUMMO!

4 ripe avocados

⅓ cup local honey *or* coconut nectar*

1 ripe banana *(optional)*

½ cup raw cacao powder

2 tablespoons organic coconut milk

1 teaspoon pure vanilla extract

Pinch sea salt

Substitutions:

*If watching sugar, use an equivalent amount of stevia *(page 51)*; however, coconut nectar is low glycemic.

1) In a food processor, blend the avocado until smooth. Add the remaining ingredients, blending until the mixture is uniform.

2) Pour into a dish and chill for 2 hours in the fridge or 30 minutes in the freezer.

THESE BABIES ARE FLOURLESS, GLUTEN FREE, DAIRY FREE, AND REFINED SUGAR FREE!

These are "get down good" cupcakes for the heart. They are made out of white beans—seriously!

The best part about these cakes is that they are totally budget-friendly and easy to make, and you will

feel great while you are eating them—and after!

White Bean Vanilla Cupcakes

Makes 12 cupcakes

1 *(15-ounce)* can unseasoned organic white beans *(Eden Foods brand)*, drained and rinsed

5 large eggs, divided

1 tablespoon pure vanilla extract *or* one whole vanilla bean

½ teaspoon sea salt

1 teaspoon baking powder

½ teaspoon baking soda

4 tablespoons coconut oil or vegan butter

½ cup local honey *or* coconut nectar

Variation:

Add 6 tablespoons unsweetened cocoa powder or organic baking cacao in step 2 to make chocolate cupcakes.

1) Pat the beans dry with paper towels to remove any excess water. In a blender or food processor, combine the beans, three of the eggs, vanilla extract or bean, and sea salt. Blend on high until the beans are completely liquefied.

2) Whisk together the baking powder and baking soda and set aside.

3) Using a hand mixer, beat the butter or oil with the honey or syrup until light and fluffy. Add the remaining eggs, one at a time, and beat for one minute after each egg is added.

4) Pour the bean batter into the egg mixture and mix with a hand mixer.

5) Stir in the dry baking powder mixture and beat the batter on high for 1 minute, until smooth. Pour into lined cupcake tins almost to the top and bake for 25 to 30 minutes.

6) For the best flavor, let the cupcakes sit overnight before frosting. Frost with Whipped Coconut Cream (page 280), and serve.

Whipped Coconut Cream

Makes about 1¾ cups

COCONUT MILK MAKES A whipped cream just as thick and rich as whipping cream, if not more! The only difference in preparation is to remember to put the coconut milk in the fridge long enough to chill. An additional plus is that whipped coconut cream does not break down the way dairy does. This whipped cream can be covered and stored for up to a few days without separation taking place. That alone makes it a better option in my book!

1 *(14-ounce)* can coconut milk

2 tablespoons organic powdered sugar

½ teaspoon pure vanilla extract

1 teaspoon matcha powder, 1 tablespoon cocoa powder, *or* 2 tablespoons pomegranate juice

1) Place the can of coconut milk and a mixing bowl in the fridge overnight. (You want them both chilled before using them.) Place the beaters from your handheld in the freezer for a few minutes before using.

2) Open the can and remove all the solid coconut cream (leaving about ¼ can of coconut water). Mix the cream in the chilled bowl with the chilled beaters until fluffy, about 3 minutes. Mix in the powdered sugar, the vanilla extract, and the matcha powder, cocoa powder, or pomegranate juice.

3) Use to frost White Bean Vanilla Cupcakes or as desired.

Vegan Creme Caramel

Makes 2 servings

THIS IS MY version of flan and it's yummy. I use agar-agar, a sea veggie, as a replacement for gelatin. I was first introduced to agar-agar while healing and learning the macrobiotic way of cooking. Agar-agar is great because it contains trace minerals and amino acids.

2 tablespoons maple syrup

2 tablespoons finely ground coconut sugar

¼ teaspoon lemon juice or white vinegar

1½ cups almond milk

¾ cup full-fat coconut milk

3 tablespoons maple syrup

2 tablespoons arrowroot powder

¾ teaspoon agar-agar

2 teaspoons pure vanilla extract

1) In a small saucepan, combine the maple syrup, coconut sugar, and lemon juice or white vinegar. Heat over medium heat, stirring regularly until it starts to boil. Allow to boil for about 30 seconds, keeping an eye on it to make sure it doesn't burn. Quickly remove from the heat and divide the caramel into four small ramekins. Be sure to spread the caramel evenly in the bottom. Set aside and let them cool for at least 20 minutes.

2) In a medium saucepan, combine the almond milk, coconut milk, and maple syrup. Add the arrowroot powder and agar-agar and whisk to dissolve. Heat over medium heat, whisking constantly until it thickens (usually just before boiling). Once it has thickened, remove from the heat, stir in the vanilla extract, and whisk again.

3) Cover the saucepan with a lid and let it cool for about 15 minutes. When cool, pour it into the ramekins over the caramel. Once you've added the creme to the caramel, let it cool for another 15 minutes before transferring to the refrigerator. Refrigerate for at least 8 hours so the creme caramel will thicken and slightly harden.

Apple-Kuzu Drink

Makes 2 servings

MY GIRLS LOVE THIS HOT
cocoa replacement, and so do I.
The combination of apples and
kuzu root calms the nervous system
and the intestines. Known to calm
hyperactive children, this is a must
for all mamas and papas! This
apple-kuzu drink is also known to
fight fevers in children as well as
adults. If my girls start to come
down with something, I serve up
this little drink in a jiffy.

1 cup organic unstrained apple juice

1 tablespoon kuzu root, diluted in 1½ cups cold water

1) Bring the apple juice to just under a boil, and then pour in the diluted kuzu root, stirring constantly to avoid lumps.

2) Serve in tiny coffee or teacups—carefully, because it's HOT!

Berry Cobbler

Makes 4 to 6 servings

Y'ALL KNOW I love me some berries, and this is my go-to summer dessert.

FOR THE FILLING:

7 to 8 cups mixed berries

Grapeseed oil cooking spray

3 tablespoons local honey *or* maple syrup*

2 tablespoons arrowroot powder

1 tablespoon lemon juice

FOR THE TOPPING:

1 cup almond flour

⅔ cup shredded coconut

1 cup roughly chopped pecans

¾ cup finely ground coconut sugar

½ teaspoon sea salt

4 tablespoons coconut oil

2 tablespoons maple syrup *(optional)*

Substitution:

*If watching sugar, use an equivalent amount of stevia (page 51).

1) Preheat the oven to 350°F. Spread the berries out in a baking dish coated with a little grapeseed oil cooking spray. Top with the honey, arrowroot powder, and lemon juice, and toss to combine.

2) In a large mixing bowl, add the almond flour, coconut, pecans, coconut sugar, and sea salt. Stir to combine. Add the coconut oil and mix again until evenly distributed. Add a little maple syrup for sweetness, if desired.

3) Spread the topping evenly over the fruit. Bake uncovered on the center oven rack for 40 to 45 minutes or until the fruit is bubbling and the top is golden brown.

Acknowledgments

I jumped into running Pinewood Kitchen without rose-colored glasses and I knew that it would be a huge undertaking. But, what I didn't know was that I would connect with some of the kindest, most loyal, and caring people along the way. I also didn't know that Pinewood would not only be about the food that I served, but about the community that WE would grow, and in return, I would find another level of healing, not just in my body, but in my heart and spirit.

The gift to serve another human is the greatest blessing we can bestow, not only on the one we serve, but ourselves as well. I am deeply grateful to my husband Lee for standing beside me and behind me. My daughters, Bella and Lola, for serving with me, and my sister, Nicole, for putting her whole self into Pinewood. Marty Eaton, the most dedicated cowboy and ranch manager we could ask for. Ginny and David, for building the gardens along with Nicole. Ted and Peggy, you are my rocks and your faith in me moves mountains. I could never have written this book without you, Gina, helping me keep my house afloat and taking care of our family and me with dedication and love. The Robinson family—you trusted me, and in return, I trusted myself. Maryalice, your friendship is a sisterhood that I cherish. Jane Ellen and the Tomlinson family, you are my tribe. The Bailey and the James family, you have shown up every Sunday for five years, reminding me that what we are doing in Pinewood matters. Heather Muro, you are my family, and your ability to witness my journey through the lens is magic. Michael, your food photography is insane, and Kirkland, your loving eye via the camera has gifted memories for us all. Jake Stearns, you are a food stylist extraordinaire. To Risha and Katharine, my shawties. Allison and Carol, you are fantastic editors and homies. Tim Hall and the crew of *Today In Nashville,* you fill my heart each time I'm on set.

To my team in Pinewood—your commitment to Pinewood is what inspires me to keep on keeping on. Lastly, to each and every customer that has walked through the doors—thank you! When you drive out to Pinewood and dine with us, you are taking the necessary action to make this world a better place by supporting the goodness that Pinewood serves, not only in the kitchen, but in our community . . . and that is bigger than Pinewood. Those in the world of social media that share each post with love—you all are sharing the message that Pinewood is a safe, inclusive, kind, and loving spot on a sometimes dark and lonely road, and that Pinewood is a light that reminds us we are not alone. Thanks, y'all!

Endnotes

1 Li, M.D., William W. *Eat to Beat Disease: The New Science of How Your Body Can Heal Itself.* New York: Grand Central Publishing, 2019. Page 38.

2 Peterson, Jane, et al. "The NIH Human Microbiome Project." *Genome Research* 19, no. 12 (2009): 2317–2323.

3 Li, M.D., William W. *Eat to Beat Disease: The New Science of How Your Body Can Heal Itself.* New York: Grand Central Publishing, 2019.

4 Vanholder, R., et al. "p-Cresol: A Toxin Revealing Many Neglected but Relevant Aspects of Uraemic Toxicity." *Nephrology Dialysis Transplantation* 14, no. 12 (1999): 2813–2815; Pallister, T., et al. "Hippurate as a Metabolomic Marker of Gut Microbiome Diversity: Modulation by Diet and Relationship to Metabolic Syndrome." *Scientific Report* 7, no. 1 (2017): 13670.

5 Li, M.D., William W. *Eat to Beat Disease: The New Science of How Your Body Can Heal Itself.* New York: Grand Central Publishing, 2019.

6 Li, M.D., William W. *Eat to Beat Disease: The New Science of How Your Body Can Heal Itself.* New York: Grand Central Publishing, 2019. Page 53.

7 Li, M.D., William W. *Eat to Beat Disease: The New Science of How Your Body Can Heal Itself.* New York: Grand Central Publishing, 2019. Page 53.

8 Athiyyah, A. F., et al., "Lactobacillus Plantarum IS-10506 Activates Intestinal Stem Cells in Rodent Model." *Beneficial Microbes* 9, no. 5 (2018): 755–760.

9 American Chemical Society. "Sauerkraut Contains Anticancer Compound." *EurekAlert!* October 17, 2002. Accessed November 13, 2019. *www.eurekalert.org/pub_releases/2002-10/acs-sca101702.php.*

10 Kwak, M. K., et al. "Cyclic Dipeptides from Lactic Acid Bacteria Inhibit Proliferation of Influenza A Virus." *Journal of Microbiology* 51, no. 6 (2013): 836–843; Kim, N. J., et al. "Beneficial Effects of Kimchi, a Korean Fermented Vegetable Food, on Pathophysiological Factors Related to Atherosclerosis." *Journal of Medicinal Food* 21, no. 2 (2018): 127–135.

11 Bamberger, C., et al. "A Walnut-Enriched Diet Affects Gut Microbiome in Healthy Caucasian Subjects: A Randomized, Controlled Trial." *Nutrients* 10, no. 2 (2018): E244.

12 Monk, J. M., et al. "Navy and Black Bean Supplementation Primes the Colonic Mucosal Microenvironment to Improve Gut Health." *Journal of Nutritional Biochemistry* 49 (2017): 89–100.

13 Monk, J. M., et al. "Navy and Black Bean Supplementation Primes the Colonic Mucosal Microenvironment to Improve Gut Health." *Journal of Nutritional Biochemistry* 49 (2017): 89–100.

14 Bosetti, C., et al. "Diet and Cancer in Mediterranean Countries: Carbohydrates and Fats." *Public Health Nutrition* 12, no. 9A (2009): 1595–1600.

15 Rodriguez, Cecilia. "The Olive Oil Scam: If 80% Is Fake, Why Do You Keep Buying It?" *Forbes.* February 10, 2016. Accessed November 13, 2019. *www.forbes.com/sites/ceciliarodriguez/2016/02/10/the-olive-oil-scam-if-80-is-fake-why-do-you-keep-buying-it/#2516c579639d.*

16 Isokauppila, Tero. *Healing Mushrooms: A Practical and Culinary Guide to Using Mushrooms for Whole Body Health.* New York: Avery Publishing, 2017. Page 40.

17 Isokauppila, Tero. *Healing Mushrooms: A Practical and Culinary Guide to Using Mushrooms for Whole Body Health.* New York: Avery Publishing, 2017. Page 43–44.

18 Isokauppila, Tero. *Healing Mushrooms: A Practical and Culinary Guide to Using Mushrooms for Whole Body Health.* New York: Avery Publishing, 2017.

19 Ren, Y., et al. "Polysaccharide of Hericium Erinaceus Atenuates Colitis in C57BL/6 Mice via Regulation of Oxidative Stress, Inflammation-Related Signaling Pathways, and Modulating the Composition of the Gut Microbiota." *Journal of Nutritional Biochemistry* 57 (2018): 67–76.

20 Tsai-Teng, Tzeng, et al. "Erinacine A-Enriched Hericium Erinaceus Mycelium Ameliorates Alzheimer's Disease-Related Pathologies in APPswe/PS1dE9 Transgenic Mice." *Journal of Biomedical Science* 23 (2016): 49; Kolotushkina, E. V., et al. "The Influence of Hericium Erinaceus Extract on Myelination Process in Vitro." *Fiziologichnyi Zhurnal* 49, no. 1 (2003): 38–45; Reale, Marcella, et al. "Relation Between Pro-inflammatory Cytokines and Acetylcholine Levels in Relapsing-Remitting Multiple Sclerosis Patients." *International Journal of Molecular Sciences* 13, no. 10 (2012): 12656–12664; GoodTherapy. "Acetylcholine." Updated August 4, 2015. Accessed November 13, 2019. *www.goodtherapy.org/blog/psychpedia/acetylcholine.*

21 Zhuang, Cun, et al. "US7214778B2–Glycoprotein with Anti-Diabetic, Anti-Hypertensive, Anti-Obesity and Antihyperlipidemic Effects from *Grifola Frondosa,* and a Method for Preparing Same." Date of patent: May 8, 2007. *patents.google.com/patent/US72 14778B2/en.*

22 Penn State College of Agricultural Sciences. "52nd Annual Mushroom Industry Conference- Proceedings." Accessed November 13, 2019. *plantpath.psu.edu/mushroom-industry-conference/52-mushroom-industry-conference.*

23 Adams, PhD, Case. "Mushroom Lowers PSA in Prostate Cancer Men." *The Journal of Plant Medicines.* February 15, 2016. Accessed November 13, 2019. plantmedicines.org/mushroom-psa-prostate-cancer/; Varshney, J., et al. "White Button Mushrooms Increase Microbial Diversity and Accelerate the Resolution of Citrobacter Rodentium Infection in Mice." *Journal of Nutrition* 143, no. 4 (2013): 526–532.

24 Varshney, J., et al. "White Button Mushrooms Increase Microbial Diversity and Accelerate the Resolution of Citrobacter Rodentium Infection in Mice." *Journal of Nutrition* 143, no. 4 (2013): 526–532.

25 Lee, Y. K., et al. "Kiwifruit (*Actinidia Deliciosa*) Changes Intestinal Microbial Profile." *Microbial Ecology in Health and Disease* 23 (2012).

26 Li, M.D., William W. *Eat to Beat Disease: The New Science of How Your Body Can Heal Itself.* New York: Grand Central Publishing, 2019.

27 Riboli, E., et al. "European Prospective Investigation into Cancer and Nutrition (EPIC): Study Populations and Data Collection." *Public Health Nutrition* 5, no. 6B (2002): 1113–24.

28 Riboli, E., et al. "European Prospective Investigation into Cancer and Nutrition (EPIC): Study Populations and Data Collection." *Public Health Nutrition* 5, no. 6B (2002): 1113–24.

29 Farvid, Maryam Sadat, et al. "Fruit and Vegetable Consumption and Breast Cancer Incidence: Repeated Measures over 30 Years of Follow-Up: Fruit and Vegetable Consumption and Breast Cancer." *International Journal of Cancer* 144, no. 5 (2018).

30 Li, M.D., William W. *Eat to Beat Disease: The New Science of How Your Body Can Heal Itself.* New York: Grand Central Publishing, 2019.

31 Li, M.D., William W. *Eat to Beat Disease: The New Science of How Your Body Can Heal Itself.* New York: Grand Central Publishing, 2019.

32 Li, M.D., William W. *Eat to Beat Disease: The New Science of How Your Body Can Heal Itself.* New York: Grand Central Publishing, 2019.

33 Mayo Clinic Staff. "Alpha-Gal Syndrome." Mayo Clinic. Accessed November 13, 2019. *www.mayoclinic.org/diseases-conditions /alpha-gal-syndrome/symptoms-causes/syc-20428608.*

34 University of Maryland Medical Center. "Largest Study Ever Finds That One Out Of Every 133 Americans May Have Celiac Disease." *ScienceDaily.* February 12, 2003. Accessed November 13, 2019. *www.sciencedaily.com/releases/2003/02/030212073309 .htm.*

Mee McCormick is a Real Food maven, community food advocate, a restauranteur, a rancher, a mother, and the author of *My Kitchen Cure: How I Cooked My Way Out of Chronic Autoimmune Disease with Whole Foods and Healing Recipes*. When Mee isn't running her restaurant, Pinewood Kitchen & Mercantile, or working on her biodynamic farm outside of Nashville, she is touring the country as a speaker and community kitchen organizer. She has appeared on national and local TV, on radio and in print nationwide. She is a regular on-air contributor to *Today In Nashville* and a vital part of the Nashville restaurant scene.

Visit:
pinewoodkitchenandmercantile.com.

Facebook:
www.facebook.com/MeeeMcCormick/

Instagram:
www.instagram.com/meeemccormick/

Index

Note; *c* indicates a chart; *p*, a picture